Starting at the Finish Line

Starting at the Finish Line

My Cancer Partner, Perspective and Preparation

Matthew S. Newman

ISBN-13: 9781515016748
ISBN-10: 1515016749
Library of Congress Control Number: 2017918328
CreateSpace Independent Publishing Platform
North Charleston, South Carolina

This book was written for Rebecca, Luke, Jake, and Lola

"The truth is, you and I are in control of only two things: How we prepare for what might happen, and how we respond to what just happened. The moment when things do actually happen belongs to God."

– DEVON FRANKLIN (CONVERSATION WITH OPRAH WINFREY)

Table of Contents

Introduction

Tenacious, focused, competitive, relentless and confident
are just a few words which describe Matt Newman.
Oh yeah ... he's also a salesman, a really good salesman.
A dedicated husband, father and son are also among
the many ways which help identify Matt Newman.

I remember the day I spoke with him shortly after the cancer
diagnosis. Listening to him at a time when most of us would
be afraid of what he was facing I only heard determination
... he told me " I'll beat this" and I knew he would.

Matt raised the bar for all who worked with him.
He made everyone better. I have been blessed to
have had the opportunity to work with a few really
talented sales people but none better than Matt. This
book tells the story of how one young man faced a
very tough disease and proved he was tougher.

– Jim McInnis, President RDR Consulting Inc.

Part 1: Preparation

One

"Why can't I sleep? Why can't I speak? Why does my head hurt all the time?" Enough was enough. It was time to see what was causing this issue and address it. I wanted to diagnose it, fix it, and move on. I had been continually told it was a sinus infection. I no longer believed that was the case. My wife, Rebecca, was shopping at the King of Prussia mall when she got my call. I told her I had a one of those stroke-type things, again, at my meeting. I was presenting when I felt the hot flash coming on, and at this point I knew what was coming next. She knew something was wrong at that moment, and so did I. She told me to meet her at Capital Health Hospital.

Almost two hours later, I met my wife in front of the hospital. We walked in and headed to the emergency room. We met with a doctor, and I told her my issues. I told her about the car accident I had been in, and about how ever since then I was experiencing intense headaches and lack of sleep. I had also experienced what I believed to be eleven or more strokes that affected my speech. Rebecca believed the accident had done something to my head. Our friend, Karen Mancini, had been in a similar car accident and was taken to the hospital just to make sure everything was all right. The doctor found a brain aneurism, immediately performed surgery, and told her to send flowers to the person who hit her because they had actually saved her life. My wife continually mentioned Karen's story to me after my car accident.

When I was admitted to the emergency room, the doctors explained they would do a CAT scan and then an MRI to get an idea of what had been causing these issues for the last five months. I went in for the CAT scan at 3:30 p.m. When I came out, the doctors told us they saw something on the left frontal lobe of my brain. We needed more information, and that would come from the MRI. I assumed we'd get the MRI done fairly quickly. We ended up waiting about seven hours to start the process. It was becoming a really long day.

We received the results from the MRI at 1:00 a.m. They told us there was a lesion on the left side of my head, and that lesion was causing seizures in my speech. Lesion? To me, a lesion was a cut or a bruise. Rebecca was on her phone looking up head lesions, and she saw the same thing. I immediately thought it was a lesion that probably came from the car accident!

Most people probably would have been pretty nervous and scared. I was relieved. That's the issue; this is why it's happening. We figured it out! What did we have to do to fix it? My wife called our nanny at 1:00 a.m. to make her aware we needed her. Rebecca went home around 2:00 a.m. to take care of the kids' lunches for school and sleep for a couple of hours; she would return to the hospital by 5:30 a.m. After she left for the night, more tests needed to be done. The doctors took me back to do another MRI, this time with contrast.

I wanted to walk to the MRI, but I was told it was policy to be wheeled there. I didn't like it, but I did what I had to do. The woman who was going to push me down grabbed my chart after I got in the wheelchair and said, "OK, Mr. Newman, we are going to do an MRI/MRA to see the size and status of your brain tumor."

I turned my head, looked at the woman, and said, "It's a lesion."

That was the moment I was told that I had brain cancer at thirty-nine years old. Life had changed.

Two

I had just graduated from the University of Delaware. I loved every second of being there. I made a lot of friends and had a great college experience. I was standing in my cap and gown at graduation, walking over to see my parents, grandparents, and the rest of my family. They were so proud. This was a really special day.

When my father, who is a financial planner, asked me what I was going to do next, I told him I was going to start working with him. "It is time for us to go into business together," I said.

My father looked at me and said, "There's no way in hell you're coming to work for me yet. Go learn the business on your own, get licensed, and come back and talk to me in a couple of years. Get comfortable in this industry, and see if it's for you. If it is, we can talk about working together."

I was pissed! What the hell? But, as usual, the advice our parents give us is often right. It was some of the best guidance I was ever given. What he was telling me was there are no free lunches. I need to earn it and work hard. It was a great message and an even better lesson. It took me years to understand what he was doing, but it was great advice and leadership on a number of different levels.

I went to work for Golden American Life, an insurance company located in Wilmington, Delaware. They wholesaled annuities to financial advisors to use with their clients. I moved to Philadelphia, the Old City area. Old City was an up-and-coming section, home to the Liberty Bell, the National Constitution Center, and where Betsy Ross sewed the first American flag. There were cobblestone streets; history was everywhere, and I found myself among an ambitious group of young people living in the city and enjoying all the perks of city life. It was a perfect spot for me. I fell in love with the area and the culture. It felt like and became home.

Golden American Life Insurance was bought by an extremely large insurance company: ING. ING was a great company to work for, and we became one of the largest distributors of annuities. The man who ran our business, Jim McInnis, was a mentor to me. He was an extraordinary businessman and an even better person. He taught me how to be successful and a professional. The respect I had, and still have, for him couldn't be greater. It was a privilege to learn from greatness, and I was a sponge, soaking it all up.

In my business, we constantly focus on planning for what may happen next, not what happened yesterday. We concentrate on preparing in advance. Most people need the benefit of planning after it's too late. They want life insurance after they get sick; they want long-term care protection when they are unable to get it. We persistently emphasize being there when things are bad, having a strategy in place, and being prepared.

This job was something I took to naturally. It started to seem more like a career than a job to me. Creating relationships, earning trust…this became a passion. It became my craft. Within two years, I knew I would never go into business with my father. I found something I loved that I was good at and wanted to do every day. I had found my professional calling, and I was going to continue to get better.

In 2000, I moved to Connecticut for a promotion. I was covering three states, and I was on the road all the time and closing business. Every day, I thought about moving back to Philadelphia. I may have grown up outside New York City in the North Jersey suburbs, but home was the City of Brotherly Love. My heart was there. I missed it. My goal was to work hard, make a name for myself, and have the opportunity to move back to Philadelphia. Connecticut was temporary, a means to an end for me.

In 2001, I moved back to my old neighborhood in Philadelphia. It felt like I never left. I lived in a city I loved, and worked in New Jersey. My business was doing really well. In 2002 I became the top producer in my company, and over the the years would continue to break my own sales records year after year. Personally, I created a great group of friends. Friends who all lived in my same neighborhood, friends I knew would always be there for me if I needed them. Everything was going the way I had hoped. Life was good.

Three

Marriage and Starting a Family

In February of 2004, I took my assistant and his wife to dinner in Philadelphia. I wanted to thank him and show my appreciation for all he did for me. As the main course came out, his wife said the line to me that makes all single men cringe: "Have I got a girl for you!"

Great, my assistant's wife was trying to fix me up, and I had to smile and go with it. She said I should call her friend from work, Rebecca, and she gave me Rebecca's phone number. When I finally decided it was time to call her, my assistant started telling me Rebecca wasn't sure she wanted to be set up, as she just got out of a relationship. Great, the person I did not want to call actually did not want me to call. I finally get ready to call and she's not interested?

A month after I was given her number, I was told she was *finally* open to speaking to me. How could I not call and make my assistant's wife angry? So I phoned Rebecca; we spoke for a couple of hours and actually had a wonderful conversation. A month later we went on our first date. I may be the salesman, but I was sold. She was beautiful, smart, independent, and tough. There was no way that first date was ending until I closed our next date. My life changed instantly; I knew I met the girl of my dreams. We were together from that point forward.

I married Rebecca in 2006 in Philadelphia. We took wedding pictures on the Rocky steps! And with no time wasted, Rebecca got pregnant in January 2007. That same month, we started our family with a rescue puppy named Mia, an adorable beagle/shepherd mix. We had a puppy, we had a baby on the way, we lived in a condo in the city, and life got better each day. Business was good, marriage was new and exciting, and we were so happy to start our family. The only thing that needed to happen was to move out of the city to the burbs. On July 27th, 2007, we moved to Bucks County, about thirty miles outside of Philadelphia. We rented a townhouse in Newtown, Pennsylvania, and started the process of building our dream house. Everything was going well.

On September 4th, 2007, we had our first son, Luke. That was one of the happiest moments of my life, and tears poured down my cheeks the moment he was born. I was a dad! Rebecca was a mom! We had a family; we were so happy.

Everything I spoke about at work was planning for what would happen next and embracing the unexpected. Planning for the future was the key to success. It was time to follow my own advice. Right before Luke was born, we had our wills done, began our college planning for Luke, and set up our life insurance. This was my job professionally, and it was my mantra. Having a simple plan set up that would allow family protection if the unexpected were to happen was the proper way to protect and preserve. At thirty-four years old, I did not really think I needed to do this, but I knew it was necessary.

The following year, 2008, we finished building our house and moved to Washington Crossing, Pennsylvania, a rural area with history and character. This is where George Washington crossed the Delaware. It's family friendly, scenic, and right on the Delaware River. It's thirty minutes to Philly and one hour and ten minutes to New York City. A country environment with easy access to the city. Perfect for us.

On February 4th, 2009, my second son, Jake, was born. In January 2010, Rebecca was pregnant again! We wondered if our third child would be a girl! All was going well. Life changes quickly and often. For all the excitement of

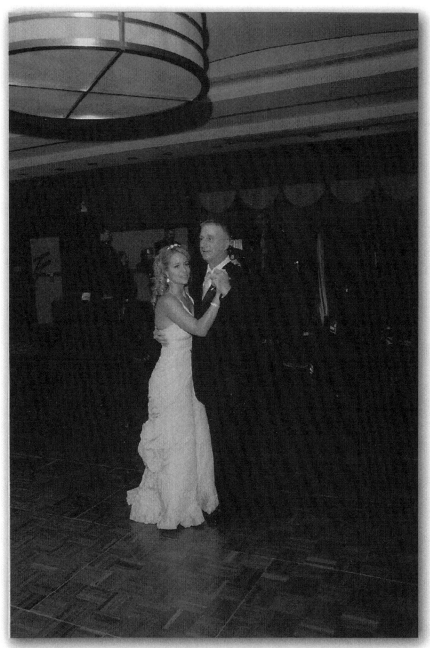

November 18th, 2006. Our wedding day. Rebecca and her father.

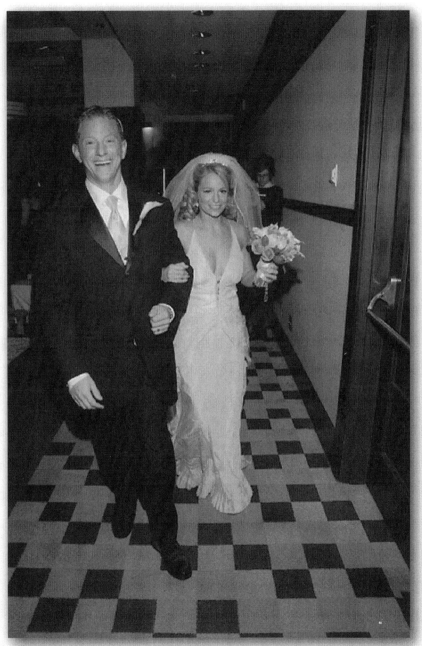

Rebecca and Me on our Wedding Day

building a family, reality and negativity would always be a battle. On October 11th, 2010, my daughter, Lola, was born. Three children in thirty-seven months. We then rescued another dog, a Rhodesian ridgeback mix, named Pepe. We had two dogs, three children, and a brand new home.

As Jake and Lola were born, we would continue to change our financial planning strategies. We were then doing college planning for three. We would add to our insurance planning to protect a substantially larger family then three years earlier. These were changes that were necessary. This was not about wealth. The amount of assets we had was irrelevant. This was about creating a plan that would allow our financial levels to insure and protect our family when we needed it most.

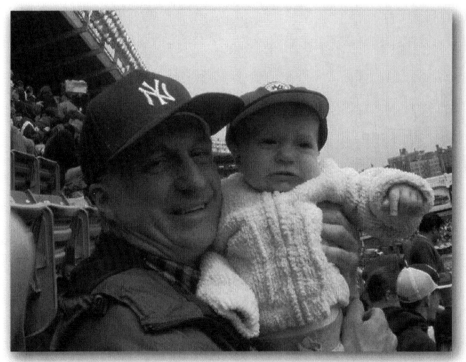

2007. My father-in-law, Larry, with Luke at Yankee Stadium.

The job of the attorney, the doctor, or the financial planner is to be there when things are bad. We have all heard the story of the shoemaker whose kids have no shoes. I wasn't excited about thinking about the prospect of something bad happening, but I was determined to make sure our financial plan would allow my family to maintain their lifestyles if life took an unexpected turn. In my mind, this was never going to happen, but our preparation gave me the comfort of knowing I did what was necessary to protect my family.

Four

OUR FIRST FAMILY EXPERIENCE WITH CANCER

My first personal experience with cancer came when I was fifteen years old and my Grandma Harriet was diagnosed with it. My mother was very close with my grandmother; they used to talk every day. One day she was healthy, and the next she was not. She was sixty-two when she was diagnosed. I wish I remembered more about the process. One day she was Grandma Harriet. The next day she wore a turban-type hat because she lost her hair. The following day she was gone. I couldn't equate or understand at my age what had happened; it just went so quickly to me.

My mother was never the same after that. The speed, the aggressiveness, and the evilness of that disease changed our family. I try to remember my grandmother before the cancer struck. That's the image I want in my head. We often remember things and aren't always sure why we do. We remember little details, and they stay with us forever. I hated the memories of my grandmother being sick. I tried to always envision her when she was well, when she was Grandma Harriet.

The day of her funeral, I was sitting in the car in front of the cemetery, waiting for my father to drive us to where she was being buried. I don't remember the funeral. I don't remember the burial. I do remember a song from Simon and Garfunkel on the radio called "The Sound of Silence." I remember vividly hearing the line "Silence like a cancer grows." I don't know why I remember that, but I always have and I always will. I get emotional

14

every time I hear that song, especially that line. It reminds me how much I miss my grandmother. It makes me think of how much I wish she could have met my children. It always makes me remember the pain and sadness that my mother went through.

Cancer made me angry, yet it also made me sad. It never seemed fair, and I would later learn life often isn't fair. I wasn't old enough to digest it all. I did not understand what was really happening and the effect it had on many people.

My second intimate experience with cancer came while Rebecca was six months pregnant with Lola in 2010. My father-in-law, Larry, was not feeling well and was suffering from heartburn. He was losing weight and looked very thin.

Larry was a construction worker, a blue-collar guy who loved to hunt, fix things, and fish, none of which I did. I grew up in North Jersey. Larry grew up in the mining area of Pennsylvania. We had two very different upbringings, yet we had very much in common. Many people have difficult relationships with in-laws. I was blessed; mine were wonderful people, and our relationship was outstanding and pure. I loved my father-in-law. He was an amazing man, and I know he felt the same about me. We loved to spend time and have a beer together. He was a salt-of-the-earth guy who made me so proud to be his son-in-law.

As the weather got warmer in the spring, I went out to play golf with my friend Rick. My in-laws were down for the weekend, which allowed me the rare opportunity to go play on a weekend! When we got home, Larry was out fixing our mailbox at the front of the driveway. That was Larry, always helping, fixing stuff, and planting fruits and vegetables for us to grow. I told him it looked like he had lost a bunch of weight. Larry was very thin to begin with, so his weight loss was surprising to me. He told Rick and me that he was having stomach issues and heartburn, and the doctors were doing tests.

I told him, "Well, you're not too skinny to fix the mailbox," and I laughed and drove up the driveway. I closed the window, and when I did, Rick told me something was wrong. Rick is an anesthesiologist. He said that Larry looked like he had jaundice, and something didn't seem right. I told Rick he just saw

15

Larry fixing the mailbox, and that I'm sure he's fine. Rick told Rebecca, who immediately decided we should get this checked out.

In addition to the series of tests Larry began in February 2010 to diagnose his stomach issues, he started undergoing several additional tests as well. Four months later, on Father's Day of 2010, we found out that Larry had pancreatic cancer. He had just turned sixty years old.

My wife had a bond, a special relationship with her father that words can't really explain. They were kindred spirits and very similar. Larry's diagnosis hit my wife hard. It hit my entire family hard. It brought back familiar and uncomfortable memories of the closeness of my mother and grandmother. Whatever we needed to do to help Larry, we were going to do.

After the toughest Father's Day imaginable, Larry went in for surgery at the University of Pennsylvania. He received the Whipple procedure. In a standard Whipple procedure, the surgeon removes the head of the pancreas, the gallbladder, part of the duodenum, which is the uppermost portion of the small intestine, a small portion of the stomach called the pylorus, and the lymph nodes near the head of the pancreas. The surgeon then reconnects the remaining pancreas and digestive organs so that pancreatic digestive enzymes, bile, and stomach contents will flow into the small intestine during digestion. The surgery usually lasts between five and eight hours. In Larry's case, they had removed twenty-two lymph nodes, which were clean.

The surgery was tough, and Larry fought like a champion. His fight and focus were inspirational to watch. He never bitched, he never moaned, and he used his grandchildren as his mission to fight and never give up. He would be there for them. In 2010, Luke was three, Jake was one, and Lola was an infant. He was going to see them get older, and they would always remember he was part of their lives.

The original plan was to delay chemotherapy and radiation until he was fully recovered from surgery, but plans changed very quickly. Unpredictability is a constant with cancer. Over time, you think you understand the ramifications that come along with it. The reality is that changes occur that are often unexpected and unplanned. Cancer runs its own course. It doesn't follow rules. It doesn't often make sense. It does what it does, and our goal was to keep up with it and fight.

In August 2010, my in-laws were set to watch my kids. My wife was going to meet her friends at the Jersey Shore for their "girls' weekend." I was planning to meet some old college friends for dinner. That day, Larry was told to begin chemo and radiation.

When Larry went through his cancer treatment, he continued to show resiliency, strength, and conviction. He lost more weight and started to look emaciated. He never gave up. After going through surgery, after chemo and radiation, it appeared that the pancreatic cancer was not there! We were well aware of the severity of this awful disease and that the odds of beating it are extremely low. For that moment in time, Larry was OK. The fight wasn't over, but for that brief instant, Larry had won. We were so excited. This was our family's moment, and there was optimism and momentary comfort. There was a feeling of victory.

Five

Cancer Rarely Gives Up Its Fight

In November 2011, Rebecca and I were celebrating our fifth wedding anniversary. We went to Paris to do it! We built a family, Larry was doing better, and it was time to celebrate our five years of marriage. Over those five years, there was a ton of good happening. Children, career, and community: that was the good. We lost my grandmother Jean at ninety-nine years old, and Larry had been diagnosed with pancreatic cancer; that was the bad. It was a tale of two cities. We deserved to go celebrate our anniversary and spend time with each other. Paris was the place for us to be. The romance, the love, and the time to reflect and relax.

Before we left for Paris, Larry's doctors saw something on his liver on a scan. They were waiting for results, and when they got them, they would let him know. When we finally left for Paris, Larry had been doing really well. He was working; he was gardening; he was Larry. It was amazing to watch his resiliency in his journey with cancer, and the fight and strength he showed. This awful disease was losing. We were very aware that the battle was not over, but at this point, the good outweighed the bad.

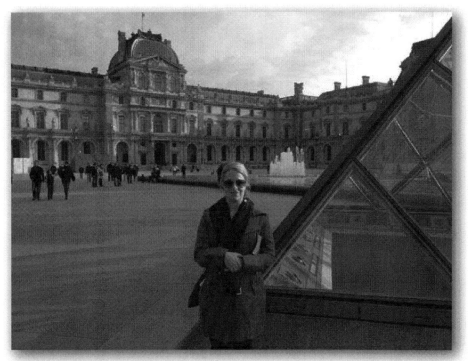

November 10th, 2011 Paris, France

The doctor's told Larry he had to get an additional test done while we were away. We figured that on our fourth day in Paris, Rebecca's sister, Lori, would call us to give us the good news that he was doing well and the tests were clean. We would then go to dinner to celebrate. Unfortunately, life doesn't always work out the way you want it to. We had such a great time in Paris up to that moment: sightseeing, walking the city, eating great meals, and loving each other.

Four days into our trip, we received that call from Lori. Rebecca answered the phone. She was optimistic that all was good, the call would be quick, and we would head off to dinner. When I saw her break down and cry, I didn't need to hear the news; I knew what it was. Cancer plays by its own, unpredictable rules. It didn't care about our feelings; it didn't care about our vacation or our anniversary. It was back for another battle with Larry.

I immediately called the airline and bought new tickets, and we left Paris. Our vacation was over. The trip back was a blur. Emotion took the best of us. Our hope and our optimism had just been shot down. We needed to be with Larry. Rebecca needed to see her dad.

When we got home, Rebecca spent all her time trying to find alternatives to help beat this disease, which did not look like it wanted to lose. It seemed angrier, more vindictive, and more aggressive than before. Rebecca was trying, working tirelessly, to get Larry into a clinical trial program at the University of Pennsylvania. Saving her dad became her full-time job. It was inspiring to watch. Rebecca cut no corner and cried few tears. None of that would get in the way of her mission to save her father.

Drive is something that's very difficult to teach; it's often something we are born with. Rebecca has the drive, the commitment, and the strength; this was the woman I married. She needed to own this, digest it, and deal with it. This was the battle she was taking on, one that, at some point, we all knew would end. That was an irrelevant thought. The plan was fight now, think later. My wife became the strongest person I had ever seen. Three young kids and a father with pancreatic cancer, and she was taking on both challenges, end of story. Larry was back going through chemotherapy and taking on that fight like a warrior. I was so proud of the effort and commitment Rebecca made to saving her father and the success she achieved on this part of their journey together with cancer. Larry was going through it, but Rebecca was right next to him.

In September 2012, we decided to take the whole family to Disney World for vacation. Rebecca and I were arguing over the cost of the trip. Taking a family to Disney World is an expensive vacation! We decided the trip was important for our kids and our family. We cannot take material things with us when we die, but the memories we leave can never be taken away. This trip was necessary, and we set forth to do it. Larry was doing well; the family was happy. We knew this fight was continuous, but we were learning more and more to live in the moment. There was much we couldn't control, but our perspectives had changed a lot. This moment, this vacation was to appreciate the now.

Larry and Jackie, my mother-in-law, had never flown before. They had never taken a trip with grandkids before. This was a trip for our family that would provide memories for a lifetime. It would make sure my young children would have remembered their grandfather regardless of what happened, and it would enhance his realness and legacy to them. It was about enjoying the moment. His health may not have been great, but Larry's smile would never allow us to see the internal battle he was fighting.

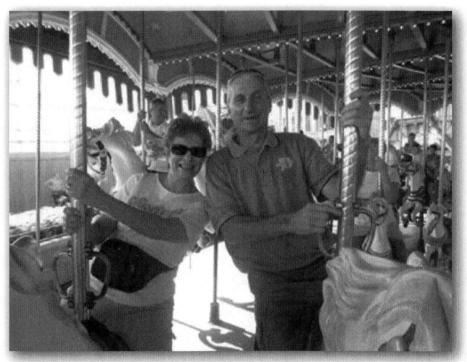

September 27th, 2012. Larry and Jackie, my in-laws, at Disney World.

Six

2013: The Accident

It was February 4th, 2013, and a typical cold and icy day in New Jersey. I was driving up Route 202 in the Bridgewater area on my way to my first appointment. It was about 6:45 a.m., and I had just passed an accident where someone had been rear-ended due to the icy conditions.

I said to myself, "Be careful today; it's slippery. Drive slow and be smart." I grabbed a paper off of my front passenger seat, looked up, and saw that traffic had stopped. I hit my brakes as I approached the light, and the car kept going. I had both hands on the wheel. I was in the left lane and was trying to turn into the left side median to avoid contact with the car in front of me. The front right side of my car hit the back left side of the car in front. It threw me into the median; I took out a number of signs that were in the ground. My airbags went off, and I finally came to a halt.

I jumped out of the car without a scratch on my body. The car was totaled. I made sure everyone that was involved in the accident was OK, and they all seemed to be. I ran to the car in front of me that I hit. Everyone in it was shaken up and not happy. How could I blame them? I wasn't driving foolishly. The car hit the ice and kept going. The police told me I should go to the hospital to make sure all was OK. I told them I was fine. I didn't need to go.

I called Rebecca to tell her what happened, and she said the same thing the officer said: go to the hospital and get checked out! When the tow truck came to get my car, I asked the driver if, on days like today, he was always driving people like me, in a suit and tie, and their beat-up cars back home. He said usually the cars, but people like me were usually in an ambulance and on the way to the hospital. It made me think for a moment, and I immediately felt lucky and thought of my wife and kids.

When we got to my house to drop the car in the driveway, my wife again told me to go to the hospital to get my head checked. Better safe than sorry. I told her I was fine. The last thing I needed to do was go see a doctor, only to be told I was fine. I had her drop me off at the car rental place in town, where I rented the biggest SUV they had and went on my way to go to my appointments for work. This accident was behind me, and it was time to move forward and get back to work!

I finished my appointments and hit the gym for a workout. My wife is someone who always suffers migraine headaches. She has chronic migraines and deals with these brutal headaches at least three to four times a week. She has had them her whole life, as did her mother and grandmother. Now I had a migraine, and I had never really had a bad headache before. Later that night I started saying things like, "My head is killing me. It hurts constantly."

Rebecca told me, again, to go to the doctor and make sure I was OK. As usual, I told her I was fine. I didn't bump my head; I didn't have any bumps or bruises. It must have been a symptom from the whole experience of the crash. The adrenaline must have been wearing off. Rebecca reminded me of Karen Mancini, her friend I mentioned earlier, whose life was saved by her accident. She reminded me that Karen's accident had nothing to with the aneurism being there, but it happened for a reason, which had saved her life. I again told her I was fine, and I'd probably feel normal tomorrow. She shook her head at me and went to shower.

Over the next few days, the headaches never stopped. It felt like a constant migraine, one that was getting stronger every day. I still assumed it would just wear off over time, and I'd be fine in the near future. Over the next five weeks, it continually got worse, and I started losing my ability to sleep. I usually fall asleep with no problem, but all of a sudden, I was waking up at one or two o'clock in the morning, unable to fall back to sleep because the pain was so severe. While I waited for things to get better, I was becoming increasingly concerned that they were getting worse on a daily basis. I hoped this was all going to wear off, but I started worry that it wasn't going to happen. Things were getting more intense instead of better. I was confused and unsure what to do, and I just kept hoping it would go away.

Seven

My First Experience with a Neurological Issue

Later that month, I was holding one of my typical "Lunch and Learn" meetings at Maggiano's in Bridgewater, New Jersey. I've done these hundreds of times. I have these events down and really enjoy them. One of my best skills is public speaking. There are a lot of things I do not do well, but speaking in public is something I enjoy that comes easily to me. I generally get up in front of fifty to one hundred financial advisors, and I speak on subjects to help their businesses, help their client's prepare financially, and provide products that help fill those needs.

My relationships with the majority of my clients are more than just work associations; these people are my friends. Many I have worked with for almost 13 years. There are a lot of things I love to do: snowboard, play golf, work out, and spend as much time as possible with my family. I love my job as well. I love having the opportunity to speak in front of groups, providing them with strategies and solutions to help develop well-executed financial income plans. Plans which will allow them to be there for there clients when things are bad, when they are needed the most.

I was in the middle of my presentation; all was going well. Everyone in the audience was taking notes and asking questions. Halfway through, I felt like a bucket full of hot air was thrown in my face; it was similar, I'm sure, to what a hot flash feels like to a woman. I could not get a word out. It sounded like I was grunting and gurgling and not making sense. I didn't know where I was. I was unaware of what was going on. I couldn't even remember what I was trying to say.

I was confused and suddenly scared. I saw myself standing outside of my body, telling myself, "You are having a stroke." It probably lasted seven to nine seconds. It felt like an eternity. I pulled myself together, looked at the crowd, and said, "I have three kids under five that didn't sleep last night; I am fighting a brutal sinus infection. Let's bounce back into this…"

The presentation went on, and no one really noticed anything. But I noticed it and was scared out of my mind. Did I just have a stroke? I believe the majority of attendees didn't realize the issue I was having because it was brief. Brief to them, maybe, but not to me. I realized it. It was too weird to be nothing, and it totally freaked me out. I was having headaches, trouble sleeping, and I couldn't put words together for the first time ever. Something was wrong.

When I finished the presentation, my good friend, Scott Bowers of BlackRock, who was also presenting that day, approached me. Scott is a long-time buddy. We have done countless speaking engagements together. Scott walked up to me when everyone left and asked me if I was OK. I told him I was fine, just tired and fighting a sinus infection.

Scott looked me in the eyes and told me that it was a neurological thing that just happened. I laughed it off. I told him he was crazy. He then told me a story I was unaware of. At six years old, he was hit in the head with a baseball bat and had a massive seizure. He had since been on anti-seizure medication for thirty-five years. He told me I had just had a seizure, and I needed to get it addressed immediately. I told him it was nothing; I was just tired. We parted ways.

When I got to my car, I was really scared. I couldn't stop thinking about what Scott had said. I immediately called my doctor and set up an appointment to see him as soon as possible. Massive headaches, no sleep, and possibly a neurological issue. I needed someone to tell me what was wrong and how to fix it. Fear had crept in.

Over the next two weeks, my headaches continued to get worse. My sinuses were constantly pressured, and I still had a lot of trouble sleeping. Sleeping in the Newman family has never been an issue. All of us can sleep, and we sleep heavily. With three very young children, Rebecca would always get upset that I never heard the kids get up and I would sleep right through it.

Now, I'd fall asleep, wake up an hour or so later, and the pain in my head and sinuses was so great and so constant that I couldn't fall back to sleep. This was getting to be too much to handle, and I needed to find out what was wrong.

I kept wondering that although I walked away from that car accident without a scratch, did I bang my head and not remember it? I know the airbags went off, but did I hit something? Was that the cause of these issues? Is it possible I just didn't remember it? Something must have happened, and I needed to find out what it was to move on and put it behind me.

When Rebecca gets her migraines, I noticed she would take Advil or Excedrin to alleviate her pain. I was driving by a CVS one day, and the pain I was dealing with was so severe, that I stopped in and bought myself Excedrin hoping it would help. When I got home from work that evening, I left the bottle on the front passenger seat of my car. Rebecca saw it, and as someone who has avoided medicine, she asked me why I had bought that? I told her the pain was so severe, I didn't know what else to do. That's when Rebecca started to realize a real issue was brewing.

Each night, I would sit at the island in our kitchen, working on my laptop, and my wife would hear me say, "Oh my head, what the fuck? Why won't this stop?" After a month or so, she had heard enough. She had continually told me to go see a doctor, and my appointment was the following day. As usual, she was right: I should have gone weeks earlier. I was doing the opposite of what I preach. I was not addressing the issue and preparing for what was next; I was delaying. Unacceptable. The following day, at my appointment, I would make amends for that.

When I went to see our general practitioner, and I told him all my symptoms: speech issues, memory loss, massive headaches, sinus problems, lack of sleep, and exhaustion. I distinctly remember saying, "I think I need a CAT scan; there's something wrong." Rather than provide a CAT scan, he diagnosed that I had a terrible sinus infection. I was prescribed sinus medication and a sleeping pill.

In March of 2013, my wife and I had just started training for the Broad Street Run, a ten-mile run with thirty-five thousand people in Philadelphia. We do it every year and love it. Every time I trained or worked out, I didn't feel the head issues. I assumed it was from the endorphins being released. I felt pretty good during exercise, but an hour afterward, my headaches came right back. I was really doubting this was a sinus infection. Things only got worse, not better.

Over the same time frame, Larry started to change as well. The chemotherapy was taking a toll on him. He was losing his hair, and his energy was getting low. He continued to smile and be inspirational to watch. I never saw him look back; he always looked forward. His demeanor and confidence were infectious. He never complained; he never gave up. The outcome would be what it would be, but his drive and ambition would leave a legacy that would grow over time. We hoped that legacy would not start soon, but the strength and fight he portrayed are what legends are made of.

He became more than a father-in-law, more than a friend; he was a warrior to me. It was humbling to watch and an honor to be a part of Larry's fight against cancer. I know this was hard on Rebecca. Watching her father was difficult, and being a mother didn't give her all the time she needed to digest all that was going on. Like her Dad, she forged ahead, took on the fight, and would worry later. The apple does not fall far from the tree.

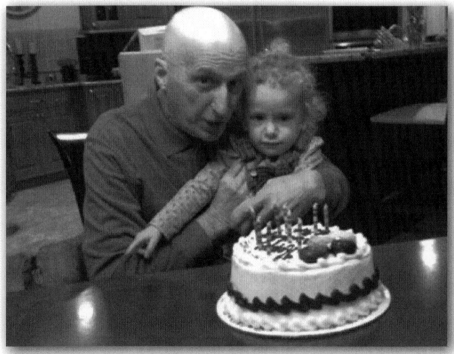

February 2013. Larry and two-year-old Lola.

Eight

Over the next three to four weeks, my headaches were getting more intense, and my speech issues continued. These random, stroke-like speaking and thinking issues would happen more often, and they became much scarier the more I dealt with them.

In April, while training for the race, I was doing an eight-mile run with Rebecca. We were running on the Delaware River Canal in Washington Crossing (where George Washington crossed the Delaware) and New Hope, Pennsylvania. It is beautiful seeing the history, the water, and the horse farms. It's a majestically scenic place to run. We were on about mile four or so, and I felt great. Rather than listen to music while we ran, we were talking to help kill the time. Rebecca asked me a question, and I felt a hot flash hit me. I was, by this point, familiar with that feeling; I knew what it would bring. While I had no issue running, no physical issues, I couldn't get the words out of my mouth to respond. Nothing came out for about five to seven seconds. Rebecca thought I was ignoring her, which was far from the truth. When I got my thoughts and speech back, I said to her, "There it is! That's the issue I'm having!" That moment, we decided it was time for me to head back to the doctor.

Things were getting worse, and we were both aware of it. Rebecca continually said to me, "I bet you hit your head during that car accident, never went to the hospital, and something that happened that day is causing the issues you are having now." I never believed her when she said that, but that day she was making sense. Rebecca is always right. I am so blessed to have a smart, successful, beautiful wife who is an amazing mother to our children. I also learned her strength and drive were just like Larry's. It was time to take her advice seriously and get back to my doctor's office immediately.

Within the next two weeks, I went back to the doctor's office. I told them all the issues: the constant stroke-type issues to my speech, the massive headaches that only stopped during exercise, the sinus pains that were nonstop, and the inability to sleep. It was the end of April, and it was three months of it getting worse, not better. I was extremely frustrated. I needed answers. I needed this diagnosed.

The doctor told me we were going through possibly the worst allergy season ever, and I had a brutal sinus infection that was causing all of my issues. They needed to up my medication to get me through this and "blast this thing out of me." I wasn't overly confident in the analysis of my condition, but I figured I would take the doctor's word for it and try her ideas to make me better.

She suggested Xanax to sleep, a steroid to crush the infection, a sinus spray, and an antibiotic called Levaquin to hammer this thing out of me. I started following this regimen and noticed it was like I was drunk the majority of the time. My will is strong, and so is my confidence, which was being tested by these issues. I was able to get through my meetings without anyone noticing what I was dealing with. The only one who saw I wasn't getting better was my wife. She knew, and I knew.

At this point, I was taking medication to get rid of the sinus issue. I took pills to sleep and felt like I was in a fog for hours when I woke up in the morning. This was no way to go through life, but if it would get me better, so be it. I try to never take medication; it's something I do my best to avoid. I wanted these issues to go away and get off this cocktail of meds, which was affecting me in so many ways.

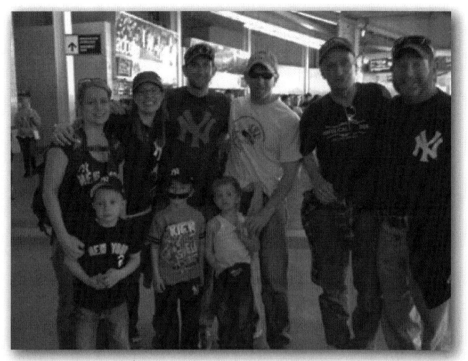

April 27th, 2013. Our whole family at the Yankees game.

On April 27th, 2013, I took our whole family to Yankee Stadium to see the Yankees game. Larry was skinny but excited. Like me, he loved baseball. To go to the new stadium, watch baseball, and enjoy the family was a blessing and a break from his everyday fight. We had a great time, had great weather, and spent time with those we love. My brother and his family, my parents, my family, and Larry all just had a lot of fun. I tried to not think about headaches; I tried to make this an amazing day for Larry and the children, one they would all remember. The reality was I seemed to be in a fight as well, one where I did not understand what I was fighting, why I was fighting it, and how I could beat it. This day was about Larry and family, not my challenges. But make no mistake, they were there, and they were real.

I didn't know it, but my life was about to change.

Nine

May 2013: Confronting Change

The first Sunday in May, we ran the Broad Street Run, and we did great! The weather was beautiful; the crowd provided adrenaline. It was an awesome day. For two hours of running, I wouldn't feel the pain, another victory for me.

May 13th was a Monday, and I barely slept. I was exhausted, and the issues persisted. The longer they didn't get fixed, the worse they got. The severity of the headaches constantly grew worse. I could barely keep my eyes open. I was on a crazy amount of medication that apparently wasn't working, and was kicking my ass. I was not me. I was making it through my days, and in each appointment and speech I gave, I seemed normal. The reality was, I wasn't normal. I could barely get through it. I couldn't pay attention to what I was being asked, and all I wanted to do was get out of every meeting I had. Not one person I met with noticed it, but I did.

Anxiety was kicking in. I was wondering if this is the way it was going to be for the rest of my life. I was scared, I was angry, and my family didn't need to hear about my issues while Larry was fighting for his life. My usual confidence started to erode. I wasn't me, and I wasn't sure if I'd be me again. I was faking it and pulling it off to those around me, but deep down, nothing was normal. I was not only frustrated, I was scared.

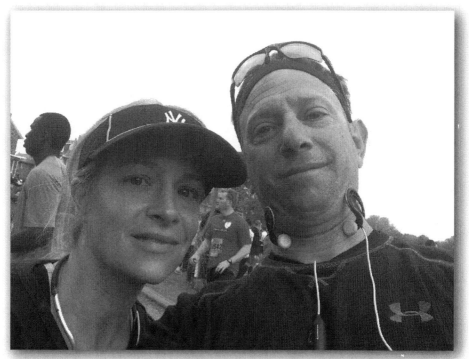

May 5th, 2013. Rebecca and me after the race.

Over the last few weeks, I started falling asleep on the couch between 7-8 p.m. Rebecca would constantly ask me what was wrong and why I passed out so early. I'd go up to bed, fall asleep for an hour, and be up all night. The thoughts of uncertainty that would go through my head wouldn't stop. I was so tired, so confused. I was thirty-nine, and I couldn't stay up until 8:30. I couldn't spend evenings with Rebecca. It was becoming blatantly obvious that I was in some kind of fight, but I didn't understand what I was fighting.

That May 13th Monday, I was driving home going through Flemington, New Jersey, twenty-five minutes from my house. Traffic circles are common, but people might not be used to seeing them in other states as much as in Jersey. You have to be on your game when you drive through them. They are extremely dangerous. I've driven through them my whole life, so they were commonplace to me. I was on the phone with a client, driving through the circle, and I saw a car driving wildly. I moved to the side, and a hot flash hit me, along with the stroke-like speech thing again. My motor skills were sharp. I was driving perfectly, but nothing but slurring gibberish came out of my mouth.

What could this be? There is no way this was a sinus infection. I needed to get to a hospital or something! I literally just drove perfectly, yet I couldn't speak or put a thought together. It hit me that there were most likely neurological issues that needed to be addressed, and my conversation with Scott Bowers crept back into my thoughts. The only issue was I had speeches all week, big, important ones for my business. I had to do them, and the following week I would absolutely deal with this.

It was the end of the day, May 13th. I fell asleep at 7:00 p.m. on the couch, woke up at 9:00 p.m., and then could barely sleep. It was time for a sleeping pill. I had a huge day on May 14th. I woke up at 5:15 a.m. and actually didn't feel that bad. I was dazed from the sleeping pill, but I felt somewhat rested and ready for a big day of speeches. At 6:05 a.m., I met a buddy I train with in the gym for a workout: an hour of nonstop, cardio, weight training, and pulling weights with ropes. I *love* working out with my friend and trainer Rob Ortega; his training methods are like nothing I have done before. They are brutal to go through, and I feel awesome when they are over. I was in the best shape of my life then and couldn't get enough of these workouts.

This exercise would catapult my day and, for a short period of time, alleviate the issues I was dealing with. It was a perfect start to a long day. We finished working out, and I showered, got my suit on, and went to my first meeting. It went great! I felt fresh, sharp, and ready for everything. I actually thought that maybe the doctors were right and this medication cocktail was actually starting to work. We have possibly found success! Maybe I was overreacting? Maybe? This day was possibly the end of feeling shitty and the beginning of normal. Thank God!

I went to my lunch meeting, which was held in Parsippany, New Jersey. It's my hometown. I've done a ton of events there, and we were expecting about fifty people. I knew the wait-staff well; the managers had a bottle of wine and gift certificate waiting for me. I saw the speakers I was working with and told them how great I felt. I kicked this thing; now let's kick some ass and make some great things happen! I was back, I was ready, and I was rested. Let's get this started!

I was going to speak for an hour, and I couldn't wait. I got up there, started my speech, and *boom*! We were on our way. The crowd was silent, writing down everything I was saying. There was clapping after various points I brought up. If, in my business, there was a game-changing, successful speech, those in that room were watching it, and I knew it. The bad was behind me; I wanted to make this legendary!

About halfway through my presentation, as everyone was eating, I felt a warm hot flash come over me. I immediately knew one of these stroke-type things was about to hit me. I thought today was going great, and all of a sudden, it changed on a dime. I knew I was not any better. Reality had set in, and optimism was gone.

Within about thirty seconds, the slurring, confusion, and loss of reality set in. I turned my back to the crowd to point to the PowerPoint, trying not to allow people to see what was actually going on. The stroke experience lasted no more than about five to eight seconds, but it felt like an eternity. I was having major issues, and the stress and fear had really gotten to me this time. Things I tried to not address were front and center in my mind. I was scared, frustrated, and confused. When I regained consciousness, I explained I had an awful sinus infection and three kids not sleeping (again). I apologized and kept going. In my mind, I wanted to finish, get the hell out of there immediately, and go to a hospital.

When I finished my presentation, I was flooded with questions on ideas and on business. In most cases, that's exactly what I expect and look forward to. That drives business. When the crowd has questions, they are engaged in what you are saying. At that moment, I just wanted to get out of there and get out right away. I needed to leave that second. I told the crowd I was running late and needed to go; they should e-mail me any questions they had, and I would answer them. People walked with me to my car, asking if I could answer a quick question. I told them I had to go, and they kept asking questions. I rolled up my window and backed out. There must have been ten people in the parking lot waving to me, telling me to call them. I was about to make a call, but it sure as hell wasn't going to be to a client; it was going to be to my doctor.

I got a nurse on the phone. I told her I had been there at least two times for this issue, and everything was getting worse. I was still having stroke-like symptoms. I needed real help, and nothing they were doing was working. She looked at my file and said that if I came there, they would have to set up tests, which take a lot of time. She then told me I needed to go to an emergency room immediately. She gave me two hospital choices that were local. One was a brand-new hospital called Capital Health in Hopewell, New Jersey. It was a top shelf neurological center, and it was about five miles away from my house.

"Great, I'm going there. It's time to find out what the fuck is causing this shit because it is not a sinus infection," I said. She agreed.

The next call I made was to my wife. She knew there was an issue and most likely a serious one. I told her I was driving down to the hospital; she told me to go to Capital Health. Great minds think alike. I was about ninety minutes away. Rebecca was shopping at the King of Prussia mall. She immediately headed to her car to leave after I called. She told me she'd meet me there, and hopefully we could find out what was going on. The next ninety minutes in the car were a very emotional ride for me. My head was spinning, not only with thoughts, but also with the intense pain that I had become so familiar with. "What can be causing this? Was it the car accident? How bad is this?"

I thought at times it could be nothing, a simple fix by the doctors. There were times I believed it would be the worst news imaginable. My mind was all over the place. Lack of certainty promotes confusion, and that's what I was going through on this ride. I was confused, scared, and unsure what would lie ahead.

Ten

REALITY AND IRONY

I n my heart, I knew there was nothing that could take me down when I was fighting for the future of being with my wife and children. The closer I got to the hospital, the more confidence and bravado I felt. Whatever you want to say, whatever you want to diagnose, bring it on! I can take it!

It was like preparing for a big game. I was mentally getting myself ready and preparing for the start of the game. The start of *my* game was walking into the hospital. The reality is, as prepared as you get for a game, as confident as you are going in, it doesn't always translate into victory. Deep down I knew that, and I knew there was a lot that I did not control. I was going in with belief, ready to take on any challenge I was faced with. Little did I know that perspective can change very quickly once the unknown is revealed.

My frame of mind was right, but it was more delicate than I would let on. I kept saying to myself over and over, "I must have banged my head during that car accident and can't remember it; it must be that accident. I should have gone to the hospital like Rebecca said! Let's figure this out, beat its ass, and move on." That was the plan. That was my mantra pulling into the hospital parking lot.

When I got to the hospital, I met Rebecca in the parking lot. It was 3:30 p.m. on May 14th. I came off stern and prepared to tackle this. We were both nervous and a little scared. Mentally, I was all over the place, trying to maintain my focus and my strength. It was time to find out what the hell was wrong with me, and I believed we would get that information that day. What I didn't truly know was how good or bad that news would be.

So to pick up where the story began, this was when I found out I had brain cancer. After my MRI with contrast, they brought me into a room where I stayed by myself for the remainder of the night. My eyes welled up, and tears started forming. I was lying alone in a hospital bed watching a rerun of the Yankee game, and I couldn't hold back the tears. All I thought and said out loud was, "I'm thirty-nine years old. I have three children under five. My kids have a shot at having no father? I'm going to die of cancer when my children are babies?"

I thought about my life and the way I lived it. Reflection. I'm a healthy eater, I work out every day, and eight days earlier, I did a ten-mile race! I have a great marriage, young children that mean the world to me, and a successful, honest business. How do I tell my parents? How do I tell Rebecca? What did I do to deserve this? What is my family going to do if I'm gone? Why is this happening to me? *Why me?*"

I cried, I panicked, I was scared. My mind was racing, and nothing made sense to me. I thought of my kids nonstop and wondered how this could happen to them. Forget me, but why them? Why? What did they do to deserve this? I had about a five-minute pity party for myself, and then it ended. I can't explain why it ended, and I can't explain how. It just was finished at that exact moment.

I wiped the tears from my face, looked up at the TV, and out loud, I screamed, "Fuck this, and fuck you, cancer! You think you're taking me from my wife and kids? Go fuck yourself, cancer. You want to fight? Let's fucking fight!" That was it. It was over, and I was ready to take on anything that was coming. If I was going down, which was not going to happen, in my mind, at that moment, I was going down swinging! "Fuck you, cancer; tomorrow we figure out how to kick your ass!"

The nurses came running into my room, asking me, "Are you OK? Everything OK? We heard you screaming!" I told them I was fine, and I rolled over and went to sleep. That was the last pity party I had, and I will never have one again. It was time to lose the emotion and figure out how to beat this thing, and man, was I ready for it. When I played sports in high school, I was pretty good in two sports. I went on to play one in college. I was a nice, hardworking, intellectual guy who got along with everyone. When the whistle blew on the field, though, it's like a switch was hit, and I was an animal. When the game was over, I went right back to the nice person I was. Well, someone just hit the switch, and if I was going down, it was going to be with every ounce of fight I could muster up. I was ready to do whatever I had to do. My pity party wasn't coming back, but my adrenaline and will to succeed were never higher. It was game time.

The next morning when Rebecca arrived, the surgeon sat down with us and told us that on Friday at 7:00 a.m., we would have surgery to remove the tumor, which was a primary brain tumor. He told me the majority of brain tumors come from other cancers. Often, lung cancer spreads from the lungs to the brain and does what is called a spider-web; when this happens, it is not good, and your time is often limited. My cancer was not in my blood, and my cancer had not spider-webbed. It appeared to be isolated in one spot. My tumor was in the left frontal lobe of my head. They couldn't tell me how long it had been there; they couldn't tell me why it was there. It was just there and needed to be removed.

The average size of a brain tumor is between the size of a golf ball and a grapefruit. Mine was 2.5 centimeters. I was trying to process the diagnosis of brain cancer, and I was going over a lot in my head. Rebecca was paying attention to detail. All I thought about was Rebecca; her father and her husband both had cancer. Life is not fair.

In the old days, they used to do biopsies to see the grade and type of the tumor. It was now 2013, and they would perform a craniotomy. They would cut a huge C shape in my head, dislocate some parts of my jaw in order to get under it, and hopefully get all of the tumor out. The biopsy would come after the surgery, not before. The news hit me like a ton of bricks. Angst and anxiety kicked in. This was not what I was expecting. This was real, and I took it hard. Fear set in, followed by anger. I had brain cancer. Brain cancer, to me, meant death.

My wife and I told the surgeon that we understood. I asked him if I could go home with my family and come back Thursday to get ready for the operation on Friday at 7:00 a.m. He told me I was not going anywhere. They needed to do tons of tests: blood tests, MRIs, and EEGs, and I needed to stay in the hospital from that point forward.

Dr. Mintz started explaining the plan of what was going to happen and where we were going. He said, "Let me tell you what we are going to do."

I immediately chimed in. "So, let me tell you what we are going to do. You're going to get this shit out of my head, and I'll take care of the rest!" I think he was very surprised by my aggressive mindset and massive amount of optimism.

He gave me a huge smile and told me that 80 percent of recovery, in many cases, is based on attitude.

The majority of people hit with bad news look back on their lives with regret and resentment. Then they see the financial position they have left themselves in and the lack of love they have shown, and they spiral down and struggle to recover. Many of us have heard the stories of the husband who dies after fifty years of marriage, and the perfectly healthy wife dies within the next year. That can be the sign of a downward spiral where people simply give up. Well, that was not going to be the case with me. I was ready to kick this thing's ass any way I could for my kids! The fight had started. I was well aware that I can control attitude, fortitude, and faith. I couldn't control what cancer would do or the direction it would go. I knew that, but I pushed it down to a place where I wouldn't acknowledge it. I would own this fight. It was mine, not cancer's.

Dr. Mintz told us it appeared I had a grade two cancer, which is the second-lowest grade, but this could not be confirmed until the biopsy. This was good news; benign would have been the best news, though. It appeared the cancer was not deep into the brain but rather closer to the surface. Good news as well, compared to the alternative. He also told us that I would need multiple MRIs to make sure they wouldn't hurt my speech or memory during the operation. If they were able to figure this out, then I'd be able to sleep during the operation rather than stay up to help ensure they don't cut into the wrong spots. I really wanted to be put to sleep. I did not want to be awake while getting half of my skull cut off, so hearing I could be knocked out was more good news. In my mind, things were going my way. I felt I was in control of this fight.

My tumor was 2.5 centimeters, roughly the size of a jelly bean. We caught it early and small, but we had no diagnosis for where it came from, how it got there, and why it was there. We kept asking if it was from the car accident, and we were told 100 percent that the accident had absolutely nothing to do with it. Just like Karen Mancini, I believe the car accident actually saved my life and allowed us to find this at a small size before it continued to grow.

Did the accident happen for a reason? Did it activate the issues I was having? I do not know the answers to these questions, but I now believe everything happens for a reason. The reason for that accident was finding this tumor. I didn't always believe that; I used to believe a lot in irony. I don't any longer. I think perspective and beliefs can be changed at the most difficult of times by the most ardent of challenges. I was confident, but I started to alter my beliefs. Destiny made more sense to me than irony at this point. I started to feel my thought process changing in certain areas. My perspective was changing, becoming better…why did it take this event for that to happen?

The focus was on getting rid of this tumor and getting back to living my life. I knew I'd never be normal again, and oddly enough, I welcomed it. I was learning lessons and gaining perspective from cancer that I never had before. Cancer is evil and it is unfair, but it also allowed me to learn from it. Change breeds opportunity. I was taking advantage of the disease, not letting it take advantage of me. I was making this my experience where I took cancer along for the ride, not the other way around. I was learning a new approach to appreciation, a new approach to love, and the ability to live more in the moment than I ever had before. I was going to beat this. I was going to be there for my family.

I'd be lying if I said I wasn't nervous and scared. The fear drove my change in beliefs. I had to welcome those changes and learn from them; they needed to be bought into and owned. It was not easy, but prosperity from change never is. I bought in.

I find it extremely sad that oftentimes people learn the most basic and simple life lessons by going through the most difficult and challenging times. Not everyone gets to keep living and appreciate and acclimate to these lessons. In my mind, failure was not an option, and I was open to change, getting better, and beating cancer and learning from it. These are thoughts that were unimaginable to me until I had to confront them head-on. Lessons are often out there, and I made a conscious decision to be more observant of them going forward. I was not only going to find them in negative experiences. I was going to get better and use cancer as a tool. It was teaching me, and I was open to a change in perspective, one without negativity.

Character is displayed during times of turmoil and challenge. Many times we act and react out of fear; nothing positive can come from that. We preach preparation in financial planning and to be as ready as possible in order to afford the opportunity to alleviate as much stress as possible when the unexpected strikes. That being said, there are certain times that we face challenges we cannot prepare for. When this happens, we put our fears aside, and we step up to face the issue head-on. We won't always win, but facing adversity boldly and ferociously give us the best opportunity to succeed. It inspires those around us to see us battle with dignity and strength.

If we lose, our spirits will be remembered for extraordinary attitudes and perspective. Legacy will be respected and revered. Oftentimes, it will be honored. If we roll over, if we don't fight, if we don't change, if we don't acclimate…we will be remembered for that. It's not easy, but we are all capable of taking on these challenges. It's unfortunate that many times we need our backs pushed against the wall to truly show the fire and tenacity that's in our bellies. When that challenge is presented, champions and warriors rise to the occasion to fight. We all have that in us. It's there. Sometimes, it just needs to be found.

The doctor walked us through the operation and told us exactly how it would happen: how long it would be, what they would do, and the time for expected recovery. The following Saturday, my oldest friend was getting married in Texas, and all my high school friends were going. I'd been looking forward to this for five months, seeing friends I had grown up with and had not seen in years, reminiscing about the old days, and catching up on the present. I asked the doctor if I could fly the following week so I could attend the wedding.

He shot me a very perplexed look. "Technically, yes, but you realize you are getting major brain surgery?"

My wife then called and texted all my friends who were going to the wedding and said, "Matt is not coming. He's going to tell you all he is. Don't listen to him or encourage him."

In my mind, I was beating this. A week from now I'll be perfect! Was I optimistic? You bet. Was my wife correct to tell them that? *Absolutely*! I was not going to be perfectly healed next week, but my belief in winning, conquering this disease, and moving on was so strong that I was overly optimistic in a lot of ways. I believed I would be able to go and just be present. I had never been through anything like this before, and I was unaware of the real path I was headed down. I didn't know the true results of the biopsy and the type and grade of cancer I was dealing with. There are many things that can be taken away from me, but my will and my optimism to be a better son, father, husband, friend, and colleague was not going to change. End of story! Checks and balances are extremely important, and thank God for Rebecca helping me to keep that perspective and that optimism in check.

I realized I would not be attending this wedding, and as much as I believed in myself beating cancer, this was a glimpse into the reality of what still lay ahead. This battle was far, far from over after surgery. I knew I could not do this alone. I needed my loved ones, I needed support, and I needed those checks and balances to make sure we attacked this recovery the right way. This was a team effort, and I accepted that. This was not only humbling, it was real.

The next morning, my family was coming down to see me in the hospital. That morning, I asked Rebecca to hand me my iPad. She asked me if I was going to watch a movie or check e-mail or something. I told her all was good; I just wanted to look something up on the Internet, and I smiled at her. I realized the severity of the disease and the operation I was taking on. It was time to make sure that if things did not go well, my family was taken care of. The first thing I pulled up on my iPad was my will. After going over it, I realized I never added Lola to it. I also understood that as long as my wife was alive, it would flow through her, and Lola could be added later.

I then went through my insurance, both personal and through my employer, Transamerica. With the planning that we had done, my family would be able to maintain their lifestyle financially. Perfect, one less thing to worry about. I went through my investments, my mortgage, and all my financial information. I realized immediately that all the speeches I do, all the preaching of planning for the bad, were all about *me*! Everything I did to help others protect, plan, and preserve was really a story about me. I just didn't realize it until that moment. That hit me hard. The realization that I had practiced what I preached alleviated an unnecessary burden that would divert my intention from my only goal, a long life with my wife and children.

A family's financial planning strategy was something no longer confined to a hypothetical situation involving statements, legal documents, and pieces of paper; it was real. I owned it, and a feeling of pride sunk in. I was who I said I was. I was now able to focus on one thing, the most important thing: *getting better*!

Later that morning, everyone showed up. My brother, my kids, my parents, my mother and sister-in-law, and Larry. I knew exactly how this was going to go. I knew my parents were a mess, and who could blame them? Their son having brain cancer is the last thing parents should have to deal with. It's scary and life-changing news to digest. I know my family well. I knew they were terrified, and that killed me. I wanted them to share my confidence, but they were on a different part of this journey than I was. I also knew the second my parents walked into that hospital room, they would be strong and supportive. They wouldn't let me see their despair, although I knew it was there. Their strength was contagious and appreciated, and it helped me look past the fear.

The support from my family was overwhelming, and the same was true of my friends and clients. They were all there for me. The text messages, e-mails, packages, and flowers I received were uplifting. They brought me to tears. Not scared tears, not negative tears, but tears of how proud I was to be surrounded by such amazing people. I was proud and humbled to be supported and loved by people who meant so much to me. It was an amazing vibe of positivity, which encouraged my belief that this was just a speed bump in my life that I would conquer before getting right back to full speed.

I was not just fighting for me. I was fighting for my family. I was so focused on my wife and children; when my parents walked in, my thoughts and feelings started to shift. I started to think of everything they have ever done for me, taught me, and supported me through. The miserable thought of them having to bury a child fueled my optimism and positive attitude. I used that drive to my advantage because I knew that my resolve would be significant to winning this battle with cancer.

I was aware that mental toughness and fortitude are not cures for physical diseases, but when I would think about that, negative thoughts and concerns would rush over me. That was real. I would gain nothing by sitting in a world of fear and allowing cancer to dictate my feelings and thoughts.

This was my battle with cancer, not cancer's battle with me. I owned my perspective; cancer did not. I would take all the negativity, all the evil that cancer wanted me to focus on, and push it to an area that I would not acknowledge. I knew it was there, but my focus was on the fight, on the victory. I'd address that other stuff when necessary, if necessary. Knowing what my family would have to go through was inspiration enough for me, and that vision was getting me mentally prepared for this fight. I also had a warrior visiting me who was fighting his own battle: Larry. That was the all the motivation that I needed.

I asked my father to come sit on the hospital bed and talk to me. The smile on his face was not overshadowed by the fear in his eyes. I felt extremely connected to him and my mother, and the masks they wore did not sway my understanding of what they felt. I understood it, embraced it, and told them I was OK. When my father came to my bed, I pulled the iPad out. I showed him my will, the will he told me I had to do. I showed him my insurance, which he also told me I had to do. I showed him all the planning that his leadership inspired me to do.

When I finished, I threw the iPad on the bed and told my father, "There is only one thing I am focused on now. One."

He looked at me and said, "What?"

I answered, "Getting better. All the planning, all the preparation, it's all done. I have one thing to worry about, and that's beating this fucking disease." For the first time in my life, I saw my father cry.

He then looked at me and told me I would beat this. I answered that I had no doubts. He then said his perspective had changed and that it was my job to make everybody aware of what I just told him. Everyone needed to know that regardless of your wealth, if you have a plan in place, you can focus on what's important. He told me how proud of me he was, and I said to him how lucky I was to have him as a father, a friend, and a teacher.

I had learned how to fight disease from a warrior. I had lived with and watched Larry's journey and the way he forged ahead. Cancer may have been a fight that would eventually win physically, but Larry never allowed to it beat him emotionally. The thought that I would use those unrealized lessons, his guidance, and his inspiration to find the strength to fight my own battle was eye-opening. I didn't think I would need them; I just thought I was watching them.

Never in my wildest dreams did I believe my wife would need to take care of her husband, her father, and our children as both the men in her life fought cancer. This was not fair! While Larry fought and clawed, it all now made sense to me. I thought I understood why he fought with such overwhelming dignity, but going on my own journey with cancer, I now understood it differently. Larry's fight wasn't about him; it was about those around him.

I was there for him, and he was there for me; our bond silently became stronger. It's hard to explain how bad news can inspire greatness. It's difficult to put into words how going through hell becomes a better fight when you're not in it alone. We were there for each other before cancer, we were both dealing with cancer, and we'd both fight cancer together. We each had our own fight, but we both knew that in a way, we were in this together. While we had never verbally spoken those words to each other, we never needed to. We both understood and rose to the occasion for each other and for our family.

Don't be fooled by my optimism; I was well aware there is only so much I can control when it comes to health. I was extremely cognizant that certain things were out of my control. I *can* control my perspective, attitude, and my optimism. I was focused on maintaining the right mindset. I was aware of the things I couldn't control, but I pushed them down, compartmentalized them, and focused on what I could control. It was not easy, but it was real. What was out of my hands would not diminish my optimism, not a chance. If it got bad, I'd deal with it then. No cart before the horse that day.

When diagnosed with cancer, often all the fighting and positive attitude in the world can't save us physically from this awful disease. I was aware of that, but I shut that out and focused my energy on doing all I could to fight, stay optimistic, and win. That was it; it was what I could control. It wasn't easy, but it was necessary.

I also became aware that the less minutia I had to deal with, the more focus I would have to direct toward the problem at hand. I wasn't complaining about a lack of financial planning or being out of shape. Health and wealth were integrated together more than I ever realized. Having a concrete plan in place eliminated any anger or resentment going through my mind and afforded me the ability to focus on getting better with a clean mind and a clean spirit. I got it.

As my second day in the hospital came to an end and I began to receive the results of the MRIs, the news was sounding more and more positive. The tumor seemed to be a lower grade than previously thought, although a pathology report would have to confirm it. It was speculation, but Rebecca and I were extremely happy to hear that. I was also told that my healthy lifestyle and fitness routine would work significantly to my advantage in the recovery process. I can't even begin to stress how important diet and fitness are.

When I graduated college and started my job wholesaling financial products, I knew I would be working extremely long hours and would be on the road a lot. I was a guy who loved sports, but the time was not there to play on a team. Career came first. I adopted fitness as my sport. Working out and running were on my schedule. I become obsessed with exercise and loved it. Rebecca felt the same, and we shared this love of a physically active lifestyle. For a period of my life, as a Jersey and then a Philly guy, I did maintain a fitness regimen and diet to look a certain way. I now realized what I was doing was not about looks; it was about being ready to take something on and physically being prepared to do so. I never dreamed that living a healthy lifestyle would help me so much. Many people rethink their health and eating habits after something bad happens. But if something bad happens and you already have adopted these habits, you have trained and prepared for the fight. Does it mean you'll win? Absolutely not. Does it mean you may have more energy and optimism to fight harder? I believe, yes.

I went through multiple MRIs, including one where I was in the tube for ninety minutes. It was very difficult, but there was a goal, which was becoming clearer: being there for my children and family.

Whatever it took, I was prepared to do it! That was my thought process. I went through blood test after blood test, and they seemed to never end. A few days before surgery, I was told I needed an EEG. I had countless receptors connected to my scalp to measure my brain waves. It took a long time to hook them all up. The nurse taped all of my head so the receptors wouldn't fall off. A woman came into my room to hook me to the machine and a camera, which watched me nonstop. For twenty-four hours, I was on video so they could see the results of the EEG as they correlated to my movements. The woman who applied the sensors and tape was very nice, probably in her mid-forties. As this long process of applying sensors and tape was going on, we started a conversation…one I am so thankful I had.

This woman told me she had brain cancer and had brain surgery to remove her tumor a little over seven years ago. I never expected to hear that and was amazed that the person working with me had gone through something similar to me. A bond was created, and I listened to every word she said. She told me she felt fine, and overall she was doing well. There were still issues she dealt with, but she was happy to be around helping people who were going through what she went through. I asked question after question, and our bond became stronger. I asked her about her surgery, her recovery, and her life.

She then politely asked if I wanted to feel her scar. I did, and this was the first moment I realized I was going to be kindred to many more people outside of just my family. There was a legitimate connection I was going to have with people who I did not know existed. This was real; the connection was pure, and I had never met this woman before.

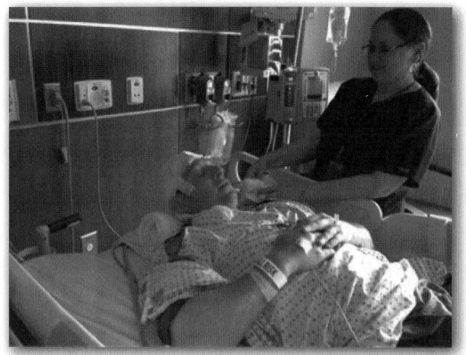

May 16th, 2013. That special woman helping me.

Everyone who goes through this arduous battle needs someone to talk to, someone to relate to, and someone who can help guide them through the proper channels of mind and spirit. That assistance must be welcomed, not resisted. I was two days away from surgery, and I already connected to this "group": those who had experienced the battle I was about to begin. I was one of them, and they were one of me. I welcomed and embraced it. I don't remember this inspiring woman's name, but I will always hope and pray for her. I always hold her responsible for giving me comfort in knowing that I was not alone, and this can and will be conquered by myself and others. I was feeling more confident than ever at that point; I am forever thankful for that woman's strength and support.

I continued to receive optimism and love from friends and family. My phone did not stop ringing with calls and texts from friends, family, and clients, who I have learned are friends as well. It got to the point that Rebecca had to give people her number so my phone wasn't the only one blowing up.

It was inspiring. It pumped me up. It drove me to feeling that cancer was the underdog, and it had no shot. This was the message I texted to hundreds of friends and family that day:

"I'm in the hospital. Fucked up. I've been getting these little seizures in my speech, for a bit, like eight seconds. It happened yesterday; I got sent to the hospital; they found a lesion, small, on my brain behind my eye. The lesion is actually a brain tumor. F'n nuts, waiting to see how we remove. I have a doctor buddy that will always tell me straight that he thinks I'll get through this OK but need more answers. I haven't eaten in eighteen hours. I'm getting crabby! It's actually all good. It's as good a diagnosis as I can get. It goes well I'm working out, playing golf, eight days from now. It's low grade and small, we think. It's as good as I could want rather then nothing. Big-ass scar coming though."

The way the news of my diagnosis spread among people I know was overwhelming to me. The number of cards, gifts, texts, e-mails, and calls of support was mind-blowing. It validated that I had an amazing support system there for me. I heard from people from high school whom I hadn't seen in twenty years. I can't articulate what that meant to me and the confidence it ignited in me. The family financial planning was in order if things didn't go well; that removed a lot of stress and allowed me to focus forward. I had my family and friends thinking and praying for me, making me aware I was not going through this journey alone. I understood that there were others like me. I knew I could do this. Worrying was meant for another time. We were getting close to the operation, and I was ready for the battle.

That evening, Rebecca and my family all left. I was alone in the room. I was in this awful bed, connected to what felt like twenty machines. When I rolled onto my stomach to sleep, chords disconnected and I got strangled and caught up. It was not a night at the Ritz Carlton. There was a time in my life where I would've been irritated and pissed off by this, but this was not that time. I was focused. I was OK. I was ready. People react differently to bad news. I never questioned in my mind that I would beat this. I would take it on. I can handle what it would bring. I would win. Losing was not an option, and the support and optimism that were given to me allowed me to be ready for my next challenge in this journey: brain surgery.

The next morning, I woke up and wished the operation was that day. I was ready! Let's go; let's go now! I continued to get MRIs and tests to prepare for the operation.

I was focused on waking up better than before after they put me under and had completed the surgery. The messages of hope and love continued to pour in. They made me laugh, they made me cry, and they made me appreciate the moment, the now, more than I ever had before. They were so inspiring to me. They were out of love. That's it. I was brimming with confidence. All those messages I received and all the visits from friends and family continued to fill me with even more hope and belief that I would beat cancer and I would win. I was so confident. I was ready. I would not disappoint anyone, and most importantly, I would not leave my children to grow up without a father. That wasn't going to happen; I was sure of it.

I'm a big fan of the New York Giants. When the Giants were losing 14–10 to the New England Patriots in the Super Bowl, Michael Strahan was walking up and down the sideline telling everyone on the team, "Seventeen to fourteen is the final, OK? Seventeen to fourteen, fellas. One touchdown and we are world champions. *Believe it, and it will happen!*" I took on that same feeling. I believed it; it would happen. I would win.

Rebecca was getting ready to leave for the night. I couldn't imagine the thoughts that were going through her head. Her perspective was different from mine; we looked at this from different angles. She knew a lot about the cancer experience from her journey with her father. Rebecca is the strongest person I have ever met. She had a husband battling brain cancer, who was about to be operated on. At the same time, she had a father who was battling pancreatic cancer. We had three children under five who didn't understand what was going on but demanded her attention. She did what she needed to do; she took care of all of us.

Rebecca knew I was ready, but she was scared. Before she left, I wanted to take a shower to be ready for the next day. Rebecca said she needed to talk to me about a few things while I was in the bathroom. It was the night before my surgery, and my wife and I shared an amazing moment in the bathroom of that hospital room, a moment of love and emotion, one that we will treasure and never forget. Everyone is scared about tomorrow, and we snuck off to have a private moment. That's us. There was no chance I wasn't coming full speed back to Rebecca. This was love. This was, and is, my soulmate.

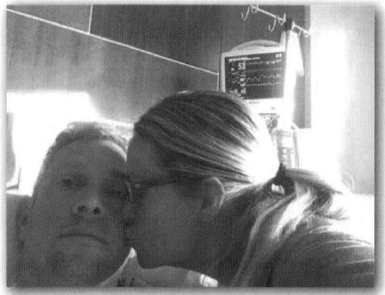

May 16th. The night before surgery.

Eleven

May 17th: Surgery

The next morning, I was fired up. I wouldn't say I slept that night; my mind was racing all over the place. Many of the feelings that I chose not to address, the ones I pushed away, made appearances. I tried to remain positive and maintain my belief that I would beat this. The truth is the majority of the time, I did, but thoughts I didn't want to have would continue to pop into my head. Thoughts of death and that the surgery might not work, thoughts that provoked fear and isolation. I was by myself, and I needed to remain focused and not get caught up in negative feelings. Easier said than done. I was ready or as ready as I could be. I thought of my family nonstop.

It was time for surgery. I was ready! The bad thoughts were no longer present at that moment. The hospital staff came to get me about 7:00 a.m. on Friday, May 17th. I was not nervous. I thought I'd be scared; this was major brain surgery, and you never know what can happen. I can honestly say I wasn't scared at all. I was prepared; I was ready.

The surgery was going to end the headaches and end the pain. When I was being wheeled into the operating room, I continually told my wife I loved her. As nervous as she was, she knew I was ready and not intimidated.

Confidence is a hard thing to fake. Being scared is OK. We are allowed to have fear. Confidence trumps fear, and when things are bad, belief in yourself will help you rise to the occasion. I had no control over the operation, but I did control my belief and my confidence. I talked confidently to the surgery team, letting them know it was time to get this cancer out of me. I high-fived a few guys in the surgery room, and then the anesthesia kicked in.

Days before my surgery, Rebecca and Dr. Mintz had spoken about possible issues. He asked Rebecca what I did for a living. Rebecca explained I spoke professionally as a wholesaler. Dr. Mintz seemed very nervous and concerned, and alerted Rebecca that my speech could be seriously effected from the operation. Where they would be cutting the cancer out could effect both speech and memory. More possible issues and challenges.

I remember the anesthesia being given to me, and then suddenly I was trying to wake up. I was hearing the nurses trying to get me to speak. I was very slowly coming to, and they kept asking me if I could say my name and where I was. I replied in a daze, "Where the fuck are the painkillers?" and I saw a nurse smile and say, "He's OK."

Many people who have brain surgery wake up and need rehab for speech, memory, or motor skills, depending on where the tumor is removed, how deep it is, and how big it is. I had my memory, my speech, and a ton of pain. I slowly came to, and I started looking for the morphine drip.

I just had half my skull cut into on the left side, a part of my jaw was removed to get to the tumor, and I looked like Frankenstein with a massive amount of stitching on the left side of my head. I continued to ask, "Where the fuck are the painkillers?"

I hadn't been given any. A nurse then appeared with the doctor at my bedside. They told us that when brain surgery is done like this, they needed to monitor my brain, and painkillers wouldn't allow them to get the proper readings. They then handed me two Tylenol. Two Tylenol? "Are you fucking kidding me?" was my response. To this day, I tell the doctors one of the best things for me in this process was being unaware, prior to surgery, that painkillers would not be an option. I was confident going in, but if I knew I couldn't take an analgesic, I would have been much more scared. The operation was done; what was I going to do now? Tylenol was better than nothing, if only barely!

After my operation, my wife met with Dr. Mintz. He said, "We got it out, and surgery went well. I believe it's grade two, but I will not know for sure until we get the pathology report back in two to three weeks."

My left eye looked like Mike Tyson had just punched me. My head was a mess; I looked beat up and extremely swollen. Loud noises were the worst, resulting in killer headaches. My father coughs a lot, and he was sitting on my left side to be with me. I remember yelling at him, "Shut the fuck up! Do you know how annoying that is?" I didn't mean it. I was just trying to recover. I felt bad later, but loud noises on my left side were brutal to deal with.

The doctor had told my family the operation was a success, but he again maintained that the pathology report would really set the stage for the severity of the cancer. The pain would be temporary, and I could take it; I had my family around me. I could not move, could not walk, and just lay in bed in the ICU. I was in a lot of pain, but I knew I'd get through it. I had been ready, and I had the support to keep me positive and focused.

On Saturday, I had some friends come up to see me, including my friend Rick, the godfather of my second child and my best friend. He had guided us through what was going on and what to expect, and he made sure the doctors were keeping him in the loop. He's a brilliant doctor, who I am so lucky to have as a friend. He's family to us.

The doctor came in and said I could start to take a painkiller called fentanyl. Rebecca and I like the show *Intervention*, and we remembered an episode of a girl addicted to fentanyl, so we knew how strong it is. I was happy! I noticed Rick had a smile on his face. I tried to look to my left and said, "What?" He said, while smiling, that fentanyl was a strong painkiller that would help. I again said, "What?"

He then told me it would only last for ten minutes. I'd then have to wait four hours for another dose. He was dead on. Ten minutes of relief, four hours of pain.

I was still in the ICU, but twenty-four hours after surgery, I asked the doctor a question he did not expect to get. I asked him when I could go home and see my children. He laughed and then said I'd have to pass a rehab test first, and someone would have to come in to see if I could walk and climb steps. I was going to have to show that I was able to leave.

I looked at him and asked if we could do that right away.

The nurse showed up with a wheelchair, to which I said, "Get that thing out of here. I can walk." I was ambitious, confident, and perhaps a tad cocky and cursing too much, but that's what worked for me. The light at the end of the tunnel for me was getting home, sleeping in my bed, and seeing my kids and dogs. I walked down the hallway attached to countless machines. I then walked up steps. The nurse then told the doctor I had passed all her tests.

I was so excited. Get me out of here; let me go home! I have always heard the expression "home is where the heart is," and it made total sense to me then.

The doctor then said, "You're in ICU; you can't go home today, but if you do it tomorrow, we will let you go home." In my mind, all that meant was one more day. Forty-eight hours after brain surgery and tumor removal, I would be home. Now I was excited! I was banged up and confident!

Part 2: Perspective

Twelve

My second day after surgery was a success. Was I beat up? Yes. Was I in pain? Yes? Did I think I'd be home the next day? Absolutely! I couldn't wait to see those three kids. Luke, Jake, and Lola were all I thought about! They were going to see their daddy, who would smile and tell them he just had a boo-boo, and he was back for good. My mindset was, "Am I going to let these kids grow up without a father? Not a chance. Cancer; you picked the wrong dude to fight with." We had no test results and no definitive reports on my condition, but mentally I felt like I had already won.

I had to win; there was a lot I had left to do. I had to teach my boys how to be men and tell Lola every day that she is a princess, my princess. I had to educate them to be responsible, hard-working adults who never give up. I've taught that since the day they were born, and I had way more to share. I was beyond excited to see them, heal this boo-boo, and appreciate them and the time we spend together more.

The second night, I barely slept. Every time I fell asleep, I'd wake up and look at the clock, and only three minutes had gone by. I was by myself in a shitty little hospital bed, connected to countless machines, and I couldn't sleep. Every hour I got blood tests and IV changes. It went on forever.

Where many would be tired and cranky, I focused on my next test to leave the hospital. I was going to do whatever they needed to get me home to my couch, my bed, my TV, and most importantly, to my kids. When Rebecca came in the morning, I was ready. I passed the tests, and they said, "You are going home today." I told them that I was going to bounce right back, and I thanked them for everything.

After all the paperwork, testing, and formalities, at about 4:00 p.m., they let me leave. The surgery was Friday at 7:00 a.m.; Sunday at 4:00 p.m., I was free to go home! Rebecca got the car that I parked at the hospital six days earlier, and we were on our way home. I was in pain; I looked like a freight train hit me, but I had a huge smile on my face. All the confidence and support got me over the first hurdle; bring on the next one!

Whenever we go on long road trips, whether it's for vacation or work, it's a comfortable feeling when we get home. When we pulled into the driveway, it was exciting to be home. My family was all waiting, but when I saw my kids, the tears just came out. Things were only going to get better; my inspiration was at my side. I was living in the moment, and the elation I felt seeing those children in my house, not at the hospital, is difficult to truly explain. It was a moment of emotion I'll never forget. It was real, and it was my moment, not cancer's.

I expected there would be peaks and valleys in my recovery, but I had Rebecca and my children next to me, which was all I needed. When I sat on the couch, I felt at home. When I slowly walked upstairs and lay in bed, I slept like I hadn't slept in six months.

I passed out for thirteen hours! It showed the comfort of being home. I slept hard, and I slept great. I was relaxed, I was comfortable, and I was home. I enjoyed my wife's cooking and real food more than ever. When the kids asked me what was wrong, Rebecca and I told them Daddy just had a boo-boo on his head, and every day he would get better. That day, all three of my children kissed my boo-boo, and it gave me a rush of confidence. That would happen every day from that point forward.

My dogs, Mia and Pepe, would not leave my side. They laid at my feet, they slept next to me, they never went away. I believed they were well aware of what was going on. I have heard these types of stories about dogs before, but living through it just made me so happy to have them with me.

Cancer does not define me; I define me! It never entered my mind from then on that there would be any other outcomes but good ones. Were there challenges ahead? Probably. Were there battles ahead? Probably. I knew my attitude was more important than I had thought in the past. I was getting life lessons from cancer, lessons that made total sense. Why did I not pick up on these before? I was using cancer now; I was learning from my experience with it, and there was nothing it could do. If we believe, if we have faith, and if we stay positive, we can take on anything. It's love and support that drive us to places we aren't aware we can go.

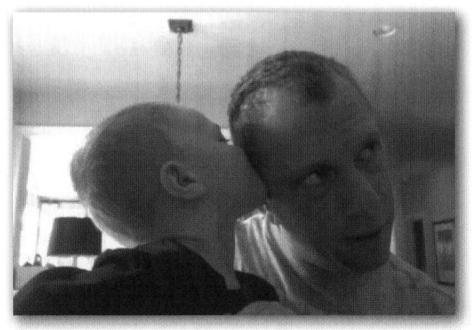

Jake kissing my boo-boo.

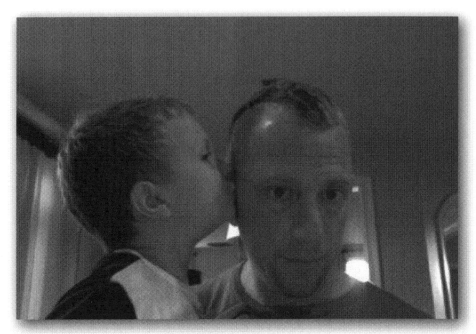

Luke kissing my boo-boo.

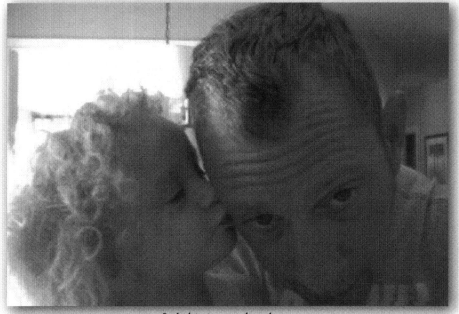

Lola kissing my boo-boo.

Rebecca reminded me that Luke, my oldest, was having a Father's Day picnic lunch that Wednesday in his kindergarten class. Since I had just returned home, she suggested that she should go so he had someone there. I told Rebecca there was no shot in hell that I would miss it! I was living in the moment, and I would share this moment with Luke. The last thing I wanted to do was sit around and mope. It was time to think about the future and get to that lunch.

I was dealing with a lot of emotion that I wasn't expecting and needed to handle. Some people keep their feelings to themselves. Some share them with friends and family. Some see a psychiatrist. Everyone deals with them differently. I started to write about what was happening to me.

My feelings poured out through the keyboard. This helped me express my sentiments and explain my issues. When I would write, it was like a huge weight came off my shoulders. It allowed me to alleviate the stress and fear that was down in my belly. Writing worked for me. I never sat down and decided to write; emotion dictated when I would do it. I started writing updates on my condition and about my change in perspective and where my journey had taken me. I wrote for me. I would pass it on to friends and family to help me deal with all that was going on in my head. The experience unveiled something built into me that I was previously unaware of.

Larry was staying at my house, as his job at that time was only about 20 minutes from our home. He was driving a truck for a construction company, so I had the gift of having him around. I believe this happened for a reason. I had someone to talk to about cancer who had a different perspective, someone who had been through it before and was going through it now. I had Larry. Rebecca continued to help take care of him during his fight. He just would not give up, and he was steering his boat on his ride with this evil disease. It was amazing to watch prior to getting sick; now it was even more relevant as we both went through our cancer battles. We now fought together and for each other.

I was on such a high; I knew I was winning at that moment and would never stop fighting. It wasn't about tomorrow; it was about the present. I watched Larry going through pancreatic cancer, and he became my cancer partner. If he could do this, so could I.

One morning a package showed up from a buddy of mine who lives in Chicago. John Deppe is one of my closest friends. He and I are big whiskey fans, and inside the package was a bottle of Whistle Pig, one of our favorite rye whiskeys. His card was different from all others. His said, "Now get your ass up and drink this!" I loved it; it put a huge smile on my face. I really wasn't able to drink it at that point, but I told Larry how great a card and gift it was. Larry looked at me and said, "I'll drink it for you. Pour me one."

My perspective had changed. I didn't think of his chemo, his pills, or of checking with his doctor or Rebecca for permission. I knew why he wanted to have some, and I immediately poured it and took a picture. He did it for me: his son-in-law, friend, and partner with cancer.

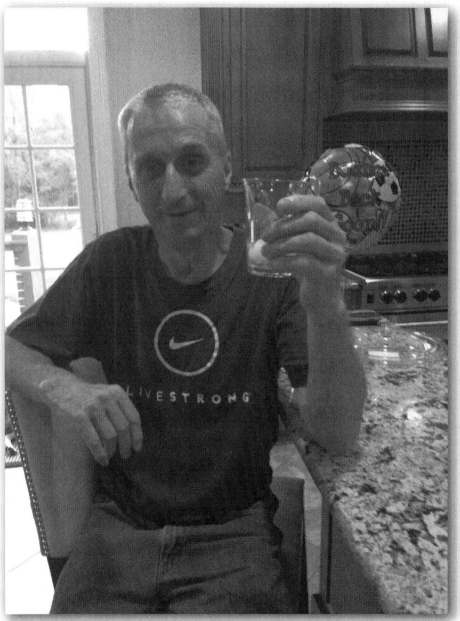

May 23rd, 2013. Larry at our house.

Thirteen

SHIFTING PERSPECTIVE

Over the next few days, I became more mobile. I started e-mailing friends and clients and began to work from home. It made me feel better, excited to be myself again. Myself, but better. Would I get tired during the day? Of course. Would I take naps? Yes. Would I feel better? Absolutely. The swelling in my head decreased rapidly, and the scar started to heal much quicker than I anticipated. I started to look more like myself four days after surgery. The comfort of being home and the contact among friends and family helped me get back to being me.

The fifth day after my surgery, I went to drop the kids off at school with my wife. I rode shotgun; she was the driver. I was tired and sore but happy. Watching them go to school at that age is heartwarming. Seeing them act like people and socializing with other kids. Every parent should experience this with their kids. Many of us may not be able to because of our jobs. Do it occasionally, enjoy it, remember it, and live in that moment. It's one that will always make you smile, and it's a moment that will not be available to relive in the future. Watching my two-year-old hang up her jacket, give me a hug, and say, "Bye-bye, Daddy" and then walk into Miss Angela's class is a memory that will always make me smile and tear up.

We dropped each child at class. At Luke's, I said, "Don't worry about Daddy's boo-boo; I'll see you later at today's Father's Day lunch, Luke." I appreciated that moment so much, and I continually wondered why it took this awful disease to teach me to live in and appreciate the moment more.

Rebecca and I left the school and went home. I had to take a bunch of medication, and it took some work to get myself both physically and mentally ready for the Father's Day picnic. Before we left, my wife told me if I was not OK, I did not have to go and should stay home and relax. "Just worry about getting better," she said to me. I knew she was right; that was the most important thing. As right as she was, my mind was set that day was about showing love to my son. I put on a hat, got back in the car, and we went back to school.

When I walked in, the smile on Luke's face and the hug he gave me would be with me forever. This was his day. His dad was there for him, and that's all that mattered. I walked around, talked to parents, and had lunch on the grass with him. The other dads, the ones I didn't know, had no idea I had an operation five days before because I was wearing a hat. When one father asked me when my operation was, I said, "Last Friday." He literally almost choked.

I told him I felt great, and being there for my boy was the only thing that mattered to me that day. I told him my perspective had changed. I couldn't explain it, and unless you actually go through it, you couldn't understand it. I wish I didn't have to go through this, but I had been blessed with a different view of what's important. This man, who I had never met before, started crying, and after five minutes of talking, he told me I inspired him, and he thanked me.

I wasn't expecting that reaction and wasn't sure how to react myself. I wasn't trying to inspire him. I just spoke with a new perspective and had great clarity on what mattered and what didn't. That conversation helped me realize how my change in outlook could help others focus on who and what are important and how we can show those close to us how much we love them.

It was an amazing day. I couldn't stop smiling. I watched other dads who were nonstop on their Blackberries and iPhones. That was me before cancer. In fact, probably more so than what they were doing. I was a workaholic and never put down my phone. Not today. This was Luke's day with his dad. I left my phone in the car.

My new perspective was becoming clearer. There would never be another Father's Day picnic for five-year-old Luke at this school again. I was there for him and with him. The lesson I learned is that work is extremely important, as is providing for our families, but there are points in times we will never get back. Enjoy them. Celebrate them. These moments are way more important than any paycheck.

I realized then that things were different; they were better. I'd be better at work than I've ever been, but these were experiences I was going to enjoy. Personal moments that I would put before other things because they are what life is about. I may have inspired others that day, but my son is the one who inspired me.

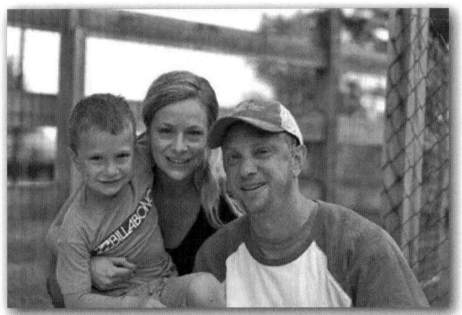

Father's Day lunch at Luke's school.

When we got home, I felt euphoric. It started to hit me what a learning experience this was. I wanted to obtain a standard of living by continuing to be the best in my industry at what I do, but also making sure I was at all the special moments of my children's lives and living in the moment during them. To show up physically and not be there mentally because my iPhone was buzzing was unacceptable.

Here was the lesson: I can do both! And so can everyone. Every time I tried to interpret this perspective change, it started to become simpler and make more sense. It was easy. Why did I not think of this before? Why did it take this awful event to make me realize the most simple and important principle is to live in the moment and appreciate my loved ones? To own those moments when they happen, and carry them with me going forward.

Luke's Father's Day lunch was a day of clarity and love, but it wasn't over. My outlook was so positive. I was happy and appreciative of so much. I wondered why I hadn't understood this before cancer, but that was a thought for another day. This day was about the now.

Larry was not currently on chemotherapy and was doing well. Rebecca had her men home, and the vibe was positive. There were hurdles ahead, but we lived in the moment, and that moment of victory was ours. No one deserved it more than Rebecca. The support and the sacrifice she dealt with was epic. We deserved this; it had been a long three years for all of us.

Later that day, Larry got a phone call from the hospital. He had a stoic look and gave mild responses while speaking. When we asked him what happened, he told us that his count was rising again, and he needed to go back on chemotherapy. This was a punch in the face, and it hit Rebecca the hardest. Life is not fair. We had such a short period of time to rejoice that we were both doing well; then the phone rang, and all the joy was sucked out of us.

Why? This was our moment! Life is cruel, and the pain it put on Rebecca and our family was devastating. Cancer didn't care that we were happy and that this moment was our family's. It had started the next round of its fight with Larry, and reality had set in for all of us.

On the eleventh day after my surgery, I went with my wife to meet my oncologist, surgeon, and radiologist. When we walked in, I told them I had three questions for them. My first question: "When can I get back in the gym and work out?"

The doctor told me technically, that day.

I said, "Great! I'm hitting the gym eleven days after my brain surgery!

My second question was, "When can I get on the golf course?" Technically, today, he said.

"Great! My dad and I will go golf seven holes tomorrow!"

My final question was, "When can I get a suit on and get back to work?"

"Well, technically today."

"Great! On Monday, I'm back." I wanted to get back to what I normally do, so I could put this behind me and focus on the future. The doctor totally agreed; he also pointed out that sitting around helps no one.

"Get out and do what you do, but don't go too far and hurt yourself."

"Done, I'll be in the gym in an hour."

Three weeks after surgery, when we met with Dr. Mintz, he informed us that he had some "other news" to give us. He had a very serious look on his face. He proceeded to tell us that my brain tumor was grade three. A grade-three astrocytoma. Chemotherapy and radiation would be necessary. This tumor was more severe than expected. This was another punch in the face. If it had been a lower grade, there would be no chemo or radiation.

I had watched what chemo did to Larry and the devastation it caused. I had to mentally prepare myself to do whatever it took to fight and beat this disease. This was not the news we wanted, but it was the situation I was put in. My battle with cancer was now far from over, and it was being fought at a higher level than we realized. Rebecca and I were both silent and scared.

The operation was tough, and chemotherapy and radiation were the next hurdle. Deep down, I think I expected it, but as reality set in, I had an understanding that this battle was going to be a lot harder than I had hoped or anticipated. I met with my radiation doctors, and I learned about a mask that would be made for me that I would wear in the radiation sessions.

I zoned out and tried to take in the news. Rebecca really paid attention to the details of what was coming and how we could be prepared. I tried to stay in the now, but my mind wandered. Chemotherapy and radiation were next on the agenda. I digested it, processed it, and got mentally prepared.

I'd fight as hard as I could, but the severity of what I was dealing with was tougher to deal with than I wanted it to be. I could handle this; deep down I knew that. I then realized what really hurt me. Rebecca already had a father and husband with cancer, and now both would be undergoing chemotherapy. This tested our positivity, but that optimism was ours; we would not let cancer take it. We controlled it, and we would not give it away.

That next day I went back to the gym. Exercise felt so good! It is a passion of mine; to be back to what I love to do was a milestone. I wore a baseball hat to cover my scar. I was lifting light weight, just enjoying the moment and appreciating the accomplishment, when a guy I regularly saw at the gym approached me.

He asked if I was training for a competition. "You look shredded," he said. I chuckled, removed my hat, and said, "No, man, I just got my skull cut into." He freaked a little when he saw my wound but then said how amazed he was. Later that week, I ran into him, and he told me that every time he didn't want to work out or go to the gym, he thought of me fighting the battles I have and how it didn't prevent me from working out. If I can do it, he can, too, he told me.

I inspired him unintentionally. This day changed me. I started to make my conversations more real and tried to get people to realize they can do what they want if they are prepared and have the right mindset. If they have a positive attitude, a strong support group, and the right intestinal fortitude, they can achieve their goals

Each day, as much pain as I dealt with, my spirit and will got stronger. Every time I felt down, I had the gift of Larry there with me; not only my cancer partner, but now my chemo partner as well. I would be starting my chemo journey the following week. We were bonding in a way that was pure and true. It can't be replicated or forged. We cared so much about our family, and the support we had for each other was something that couldn't be taught. It's earned through love and dedication.

My mother and father are wonderful people. My goal was always to be parents like they have been to me, and I am forever appreciative of how much they sacrificed for our family and how much they have taught my brother and me. The relationship with Larry was different.

When our journey together with cancer began, Larry and I created our own bond. It wasn't as much about words, but about respect, love, and family. Cancer is an evil disease that fights fearlessly to conquer. It changed my perspective greatly. It brought Larry and me closer than ever and allowed us to have someone ride with us on this roller coaster of cancer. Our whole family rode with us; our ride together was just different and unique.

I started e-mailing people at work, getting in touch with friends and clients. I wanted to thank everyone and tell them that their love, hope, and support was appreciated greatly. I started to think about the future and not dwell on the past. I will beat this, so let's get ready for a better tomorrow, I thought. My kids had their dad with them, and that boo-boo would get better every day.

Writing continued to help me deal with the realities that I had to address. I owned that outlet. It was mine. I owned the situation. The writing I was doing was my way of dealing with my issues, which were real and unavoidable. Channeling my energy to remove negativity was done by putting pen to paper, or fingers to keyboard. I was not writing to inspire others. I was doing it for me. The more I wrote, the more people responded. I felt so empowered, so strong, so in control.

I believe the reality was that I had pent up fear, nerves, and aggression, and writing became my method of alleviating these issues and maintaining my strength and beliefs. I've written at my desk, in the hospital, in the car, and many other places. It's the way I deal with my inner demons and anxiety, and it works for me. I never anticipated how many people would read my messages. I had never been on social media at that point. I had never posted on Facebook, never tweeted on Twitter. My messages were e-mails I'd send to friends, relatives, and clients to update them on my condition and my perspective. I never realized that those e-mails were being forwarded on to people I had never met. This was organic and pure. My messages were providing updates, but that started to change. They started to become more about emotion and less about my current condition. This is what I needed to say and get off my chest.

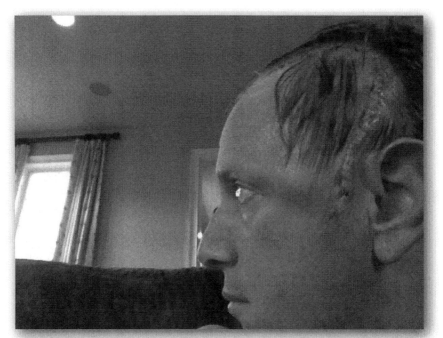

Saturday May 25th, 2013. My left eye was almost fully healed, and the scar swelling was starting to lessen from my forehead to my ear.

Fourteen

The Gut Check and the Gong

At the end of June, I started going through chemotherapy and radiation. My oncologist laid out the groundwork of the plan. I would do radiation five days a week with a chemotherapy pill called Temodor. When radiation ended, they would up my dosage of chemotherapy each month. I would take it for five days and be off for twenty-eight days for about a year. I was told to take an anti-nausea pill called Zofran at night, after twenty minutes take my chemotherapy pills, and then go to bed. They told me this would be the easiest way to manage the chemotherapy.

I told my oncologist I could take those pills right away. I was scared of nothing! He said I could if I wanted, but I should get the prescription filled for Zofran first and do it his way. I told him I was in beast mode and to give me the pills! I'll start this right now! He said, "If you want, but again, I don't recommend it." I popped the pills and went on my way to meet Rebecca for lunch.

When we got to the restaurant, the chemo was hitting me and hitting me hard. That was the moment I realized the severity of the dosage of the pills I was taking. This immediately brought me back to reality. I'm no one special; this was poison I was taking, and it was not going to be easy. I started vomiting, and Rebecca had to bring me home and go get the Zofran at the pharmacy. I laid on the couch for ten hours that day with a puke bucket at my side. My perspective on the viciousness of this "medication" was real and had to be addressed properly.

Chemotherapy was not going to be easy, and mentally I needed to prepare for a new type of journey. My oncologist had a plan to follow to alleviate as many issues as possible as I began my gauntlet with chemotherapy. I understood that deviating from the plan the experts laid out was the wrong idea. Whether it's a financial plan, a fitness plan, a diet plan…by not sticking to it, bad things can happen. Altering tactics is often necessary, but ignoring them is foolish. That's what I did. I noted them, and ignoring them was not going to happen again. There was really only one person I was able to talk to about this, and that was Larry.

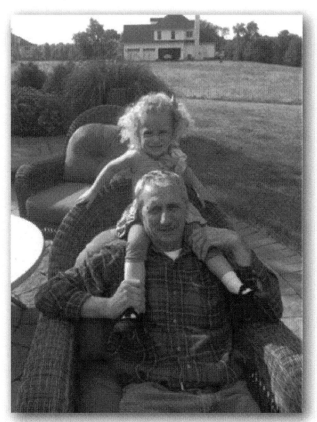

June 13th, 2013. Larry and Lola in our backyard.

My focus and my mission had all changed and become more understandable. Clarity was settling in on what was truly important. Larry, my cancer partner, was still fighting, still hanging in there. His fight was continually getting tougher. He was eating less and lethargy was becoming more prevalent. He continued to lose energy and looked extremely thin, almost emaciated. Rebecca stood by him at all times. Whatever he needed, she made sure he had access to.

When we were both going through chemo, Larry and I spoke a lot, and we often sat together in silence. Larry's chemo was through a port, mine was through a pill. Sometimes we would be sitting on the couch, and he would fade off. I would wake him up and tell him the Yankees were in a good game. Or I'd tell him that his team, the Phillies, were winning; I was trying to keep him attentive, trying to keep him focused.

For Larry, the battle seemed to get tougher and tougher, and the realities of mortality were setting in for all of us. I was with him. He was with me. We were in this together. The outcome was eventual, but this was about love and drive; everything else was a waste of precious time. Cancer may take our lives, it can never define who we are. Larry owned cancer in my book.

When I began radiation, I asked for the earliest time I could get because I was showing up in a suit and tie, doing my radiation, and then going straight to work. No sitting around and no doing nothing; I was in control. This was my life, and I would do what I wanted to do while dealing with this. The earliest time slot was 7:00 a.m. I was able to get the 7:10 slot.

Every day I would get there at 6:30 a.m. I'd have my iPad and phone to get work done, and then I'd do my eight to ten minutes of radiation and be out the door. My chemotherapy would be done at night.

Each morning I would see the woman before me heading into the radiation area. She had to be seventy to seventy-five years old. She was about four foot ten, maybe 70 pounds and very emaciated looking. I never had the opportunity to speak to her because her son would walk her into the radiation area, come to the waiting room for eight to ten minutes, and then go get her. She looked frail and beat up, but she always smiled.

About halfway through my radiation sessions, a nurse approached me and said, "The woman before you is having her last session today. Would you like the 7:00 a.m. session starting tomorrow?"

I said, "*Absolutely! I am in!*"

The nurse told me they do a ceremony for people when they finish their radiation sessions. They read poems, they ring a gong, and they celebrate. She looked right at me and said, "Would you like to join us for the ceremony in a few minutes for the woman who is done today?"

I said, "Thanks, but I'm OK. I'm going to do some work until you are ready for me."

This massive feeling of guilt and irresponsibility came over me. I felt like I did something wrong. I thought about that frail woman, and I said to myself, "What the fuck is wrong with you? Go see this ceremony!" So I got up, left the waiting room, and walked into the hallway to watch the ceremony. I saw a woman going through hell, but with the biggest smile I had ever seen as she rang the gong with enthusiasm, conviction and most notably pride. I broke down and cried. She was one of the toughest people I had ever seen in my life, and I could not believe I almost had the audacity to not be part of this. I immediately called Rebecca to tell her about what I saw, what I was proud to be a part of. I told her when I had my day I wanted her to be there with me, and celebrate a day that would belong to us. A day of accomplishment.

On July 24th, 2013, I had my last radiation session. I took the face guard that protected me, which today sits in my office so I always remember it. We read poems, and at the end, I rang the gong. I immediately understood what that meant. It was a confirmation of completion and celebrating the moment. It was achievement. None of us who ring that gong truly knows what the future will bring, but the gong symbolizes that we own the now, not cancer.

We were humbled and appreciative of all who helped me get through radiation. It was a big deal; one of the poems from the ceremony meant a great deal to me. It would emblazon my continuing battle with cancer. I may have been done with radiation, but the battle never stops.

> You gain strength, courage, and confidence by every experience in which you really stop to look fear in the face. You are able to say to yourself, 'I lived through this horror. I can take the next thing that comes along.'

ELEANOR ROOSEVELT

I'll never forget that day; I'll never forget that amazing woman I watched who I believed was one of the toughest people I have ever seen in my life. I will *never* forget ringing that *gong*.

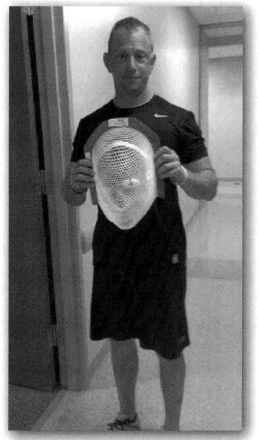

July 24th, 2013 My Last Day of Radiation

Over the next two months, the effects of the radiation kicked in. I was the recipient of a few random bald spots on my head. I lost my taste buds. I couldn't tell you if that was from the chemo or the radiation, but rather than being upset, I rationalized the trade-off between taste buds and life as one I was willing to make.

The next big event would be my six-month MRI. This would be the first major test to see if anything had grown back, if there was anything the surgeons couldn't get, or any other issues ahead of me we were unaware of. It was going to be a big test that would lay out the plan for the next part of my journey. I didn't think much about it until it got close; I was trying to ward off worry and concern. I focused on the present…the lesson that cancer had given me, one I would not give back.

Fifteen

NUCLEAR WAR

Over the next three months, I continued to appreciate each and every day. I'd be remiss not to say that as each month passed, as the dosage of Temodar got higher, things definitely became more difficult. I was losing weight, losing hair, and fighting lethargy. I would work out every day, but there were effects that were difficult to handle aside from the weight loss and the bald spots. My stomach was really messed up. It constantly hurt. Going to the bathroom became a brutal and painful experience; from my view, it was the worst part of the treatments. I would not be able to go until I was so backed up it had to come out. It then felt like a brick was being forced through a three-inch-wide hole. The pain was awful, and the experience was something I feared every time it happened.

Losing hair, losing taste buds, losing weight, having bathroom issues and always being extremely tired were problems that couldn't be avoided or treated. They were part of the deal. What never was affected was my optimism and regard of every minute with those that mattered to me. I was well aware that my six-month MRI would tell me where my fight with cancer currently stood. I was planning to be ready mentally and physically for that MRI. Regardless how tired I got, missing the gym and not working out was NOT an option. I believe fitness and healthy living did nothing but help my mind, body and spirit, and I continued to work hard to be ready if needed.

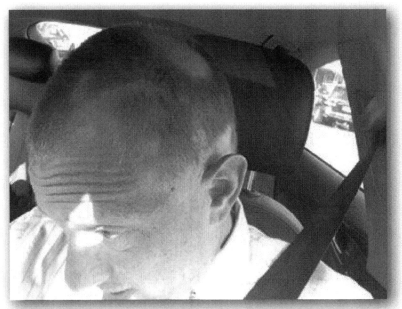

August 12th, 2013.

By living a healthy lifestyle and having a proper plan in place, it became easier for me to remove negativity and doubt from my thoughts. Preparation allowed me to focus on what was important rather than wish I had done things differently and fill my mind with resentment or regret.

Over the last six months of healing, symptoms that used to bother me started to go away. Since the operation, the brain seizures that used to give me speech problems had vanished. The massive headaches caused by the tumor pressing into my sinuses and brain were gone. I used to have sleeping problems because my headaches were so severe; those were gone.

For a short time while I was healing, I lost some of my sharpness, but that too passed and came back 100 percent and, dare I say, better than ever. All the issues that led me to find this cancer in my head were going away.

October 28th was my first post-surgery MRI. I had an MRI with and without contrast and blood tests in addition to a bunch of other tests. Rebecca was with me the whole time, and we had no doubt we were going to get good news.

After being in the hospital for about 3.5 hours, we finished the tests and went home to give my children huge hugs. We'd have to wait until 9:00 a.m.

the next day to get the results back. Rebecca and I went to dinner, and just enjoyed spending time together. We planned for nothing but good news. We got home, put our children to bed, and just enjoyed each other's company, preparing in silence for the unexpected if necessary.

The next morning, we went to the hospital and met with my oncologist at 9:00 a.m. As we walked into his office, the first thing he said was, "All good news; sit down and relax." There was no tumor and no pieces or particles; it was a clean MRI. There was no better news we could have been given.

I can't tell you the relief that began to set in. We were told I'd be on chemo for four more months, five days on, twenty-eight days off, and then I'd be done. In four months, I'd be on no medication of any kind. He told me every three months I'd get an MRI to make sure nothing was coming back, but that he couldn't be giving me any better news.

This was a great day. There would be tests and possible issues down the road, but this was *my* day. This was a battle we won, but we were also aware the war wasn't over. There was a long road ahead of us, but this moment was ours.

This was the best news I could get. I could not tell you how relieved and excited I was. To know my wife would smile, my parents and my brother and sister-in-law would cry from happiness, and most importantly, that there would be no bad news for my children to hear felt like the best thing that's ever happened to me. Attrition makes us closer and respectful of what we have. I love my life, and I will enjoy it, relish in it, and treat it with the love and respect it deserves.

Sixteen

A Change in Mission

The year 2013 was a roller coaster. We were given great memories and moments, and we faced difficult times and challenges. My wife had dealt with three young children, a father with pancreatic cancer, and a husband who was diagnosed with brain cancer. The strength, drive, and love she showed is the most courageous and selfless thing I have ever seen. Despite the onslaught of thoughts going through her head and the fear of reality, she kept our family united and strong. She is the most wonderful woman I have ever met, and the toughness instilled in her is who she is.

In November of 2013, Rebecca threw me a surprise fortieth birthday party. We received an invitation to a fundraiser for my friend Mike Goldberg's charity. I didn't even blink; I would be there to support Mike's charity, no questions asked. When we walked in to this "fundraiser," I quickly realized it wasn't a fundraiser at all, but a party for me. I never saw it coming.

It was one of the best nights of my life. Everyone I loved and who mattered to me was there. People drove four to five hours and flew in from all over the country. About 120 people showed up! I didn't look at this as a birthday party; I looked at it as a celebration of an MRI that came back clean. We ate, we drank, and we hugged a lot. We also cried. This was a night I'll never forget, and it reminded me that a support network and surrounding yourself with loved ones can drive success in so many different facets of life.

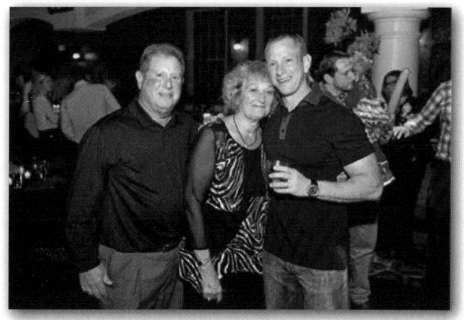

November 12th, 2013. My surprise fortieth birthday party with my parents.

The party was a celebration, but it was also an opportunity to look back over a life-changing year. I had been through a car accident, brain surgery, radiation, chemotherapy, and anti-seizure medication, just to name a few things. On New Year's Day, the beginning of 2014, I felt like a better version of myself.

My perspective had changed, my outlook on things had changed, and my appreciation for the moment had increased significantly. All of these changes were positive. The lessons I learned were real, but the journey of learning them was extremely difficult. I wouldn't wish it on anyone. The support of friends and family helped ignite a driving force that didn't let me look back. I just focused on the now. Today. My day. Every day would be my day, and every day would be appreciated rather than taken for granted.

Even with all the fighting and negativity, I experienced many positives in 2013. I finished the year as the top sales performer at my company. I had been the top performer ten times prior in my career, but this one meant the most to me. My challenges reached far beyond the world of business, but they didn't prevent or deter me from reaching the success and goals that I planned to achieve. This was far and away the most meaningful business success I had. It wasn't about awards; it was about accomplishment in the face of adversity.

It was obvious that it wasn't only my perspective that had changed; my mission had changed, too. The more I shared, the more I understood that. I was never going through this alone, and neither are others. My view on why I am here changed. I was no longer put here to just wholesale products. I was put here to share my feelings, share my fear, share my journey, and help people plan and prepare for their journey in life. I was seeing a responsibility that I owned, an obligation to share the value of wealth and health.

I never thought that my defining moment would come when I had the odds stacked against me, and something out of my control like cancer would be my biggest adversary. I never thought that this awful disease would give me the greatest lesson I ever learned in life: Appreciate the moment, live in the now. The inspiration that I have learned, I try to pay forward as much as possible. I am blessed to have learned the most important lessons and to have the most positive attitude from the darkest of diseases. That's what I took from cancer, that was my victory.

I understood part of why I was here was to support others and guide people to plan the right way. I am here to help people not back down from challenges, but rise to the occasion. I am here to get people excited about what's really important in our lives and what really makes us successful. I had a difficult time trying to figure out why I had to go through this awful experience, this dance with cancer, to learn all of this.

I try to make the most out of every day. A major change in perspective is like putting on a new pair of glasses; you see things differently. You appreciate and enjoy the smaller things substantially more than you did before. Winning doesn't always mean beating cancer physically; it means conquering it mentally and emotionally and sharing that with others. Cancer can never take your fire, it can never take your fight, and it can never define who you are. We define that.

Surround yourself with love, and you will be ready for the challenges of life that you don't see coming down the road. Through proper planning in advance of difficult times, I was able to regain my health, keep my spirit, and maintain my ability to be a father and husband. I never looked back with resentment or regret, but instead, I always looked forward with positivity.

Part 3: The Journey Continues

Seventeen

2014 The Year After and Saying Goodbye

In 2014, we focused on helping others. We started to raise money for the National Brain Tumor Organization and Voices Against Brain Cancer. We would now run races not for ourselves, but to help other families and provide tools to promote research to beat this disease. In May 2014, we would do the Broad Street Run again, but this time with a goal to help find a cure for cancer. We were a team of runners with a goal to raise money to beat brain cancer. My fight may have only been a year old, but our focus had shifted to staying healthy and helping others.

This is the e-mail my wife sent to get people to run with us to raise money for the National Brain Tumor Society in 2014:

Hello Everyone,

Sunday, May 4th, 2014, is the Broad Street Run in Philly. This is a ten-mile race filled with lots of energy and a crowd of people cheering you on from start to finish. It's the country's biggest ten-miler! Last year approximately thirty thousand people ran this race.

For a number of years now, Matt and I have been running this race together. We simply did it for fun, and we enjoyed each other's company. This race will always hold a special place in my heart. Last year, I can clearly remember the two of us training on the canal in Washington Crossing. We

89

were running eight miles that day. I was talking to Matt, and I'm waiting for him to respond. It took him a long time to say something to me. I'm thinking to myself, "What the hell is wrong with him?" Well, we didn't know it at the time, but he was having a speech seizure. On May 5th, 2013, we ran the race with our friend Scott, and we all did great and felt wonderful. A few days later, Matt was diagnosed with a brain tumor, and on May 17th, he had surgery to remove it. To this day, I'm amazed how Matt trained and ran this race without one complaint; meanwhile he was suffering from a malignant brain tumor. Talk about mind over matter.

This year we want to form a team to raise funds for Matt's charity...the National Brain Tumor Society. I contacted the staff who runs Broad Street, and unfortunately, we all have to enter the lottery, and once you're in, we will get you set up on our team (if you want to, that is). We will provide you with a custom T-shirt designed by Matt himself and would love to treat all of you and spouses to a delicious dinner the night before the race. We'll enjoy one another's company over dinner and drinks (but not too many...we have a ten-mile race to run the next day, after all). We ask if you would send an e-mail (which I'll prepare to make your life easy. You just have to forward) to friends, family, colleagues, etcetera, which will have a direct link to Matt's website, where it takes them seconds to make a donation to the charity. All money goes directly to the charity and is tax-deductible. This year we can all run for a cause, which is great in itself!

If you have any questions, concerns, comments, or suggestions, please let me know. Thank you, everyone, and we hope you can all join us. Good luck getting into the race. Last year everyone I know who entered the lottery got in. Let's pray the same happens this year! If one of you don't get in and really want to run it, please let me know and I'll see what I can do.

Love, Rebecca and Matt

Training for this run was fun and inspiring. We had raised almost $14,000 in charitable contributions! We are more appreciative of these contributions than imaginable, and our goal was to raise money to help find easier solutions to fighting brain cancer than the operation, radiation, and chemotherapy that I had to go through. We had a team of five that ran the race, and we were so appreciative of their time and commitment to running with us and helping us raise money to beat brain cancer.

The back of the shirts we made included the poem I found in the hospital and took a picture of during radiation. The poem was above the gong:

What Cancer Cannot Do

Cancer is so limited…
It cannot cripple love.
It cannot shatter hope.
It cannot corrode faith.
It cannot eat away peace.
It cannot destroy confidence.
It cannot kill friendship.
It cannot shut out memories.
It cannot silence courage.
It cannot reduce eternal life.
It cannot quench the Spirit.

—AUTHOR UNKNOWN

That is what everybody read who ran behind us, and Rebecca and I believed it said it all. We wore them for all to see; we wore them proud.

Just one week after the Broad Street Run, I went for my MRI that was the one-year anniversary of my cancer diagnosis. As usual, I would not know the results until 9:00 a.m. the next day. I took Rebecca to dinner, our standard protocol, hugged my kids like crazy when we got home, and went to bed. I fully expected great news. I had no symptoms that caused me to fear this evil tumor was back. I hadn't had any seizures since my operation, and the same was true with headaches.

I felt ready and prepared. I was up at 4:00 a.m., waiting to get the results. Our time at the hospital was brief, but it felt like it took forever. The surgeon walked in and made us aware that nothing had changed and nothing was found. This was turning into a great week. The run went well, the MRI didn't find anything, and my wife received the news she needed to hear about me.

At the same time, Larry was going through a much more challenging period, and his cancer was rapidly becoming more aggressive. He was sixty-four years old, and the chemo had really been taking its toll. Still, he was fighting, never willing to give up. The news from my MRI gave happiness and relief to my wife. I was happier for her than for myself. She deserved the good news during a very difficult period of time.

Seeing my father-in-law fight pancreatic cancer for four years when the average life span after diagnosis is six months inspired me more than he would ever know. My wife needed me to be strong, to do well, and to be there for her. I thanked Larry for showing me how to be tough. I spent as much time with my family as possible to show them I could do everything I have done before and more.

During work, I started to make my speeches and presentations more personal. I began to use my story as a way to help people prepare and plan. I was beginning to do speeches to inspire, not to sell. I started doing presentations on preparation and health and less on the products we sold. The more I spoke on my reality, the better my business grew. Honesty and integrity promote connection, and my connection with clients blossomed.

In June 2014, I was asked to speak at an event at a church. I was talking about planning, legacy, and eliminating negativity to focus on the fight that must be endured when fighting a disease like cancer. A woman raised her hand, which did not happen often during my presentations on perspective and planning. She stood up and started yelling, "Listen to this man. He's absolutely right. I have inoperable cancer. I have no insurance, no planning, and every day, it makes me cry of sadness and fear."

She started crying, screaming louder, and I walked off stage and hugged her. I was here for a reason, as was she. People saw both sides of disease, those who planned and those who didn't. We cried and hugged, and I let her know she was not on this journey alone; others, like me, were along for the ride as well.

With all my conversations and presentations about cancer and all the friends I had made who were on the same journey, I almost always saw optimism and hope. This was my first experience with regret, fear, and disappointment. Simple planning can be done to avoid this, and we need to learn from the mistakes others have made. This was a lesson for many in the room: wealth does not dictate your need to plan; preparation does.

Part of what drove my fight, what ignited me, was not only watching Larry fight, but having a partner to go through this journey with me. His fight continually got tougher every day. Rebecca made it her full-time job to get Larry into a clinical trial program at the University of Pennsylvania. She was dedicating herself to saving his life. She finally got him in!

She would make the trip down to Philadelphia with Larry just about every day. We were so excited to get him in; it was our last resort, and we knew it. Larry and I were like two sides of a scale. As I got stronger and better, he went the other way, physically. Larry was getting weaker and losing his ability to eat. He was sleeping a lot more, constantly cold, and continuing to lose weight at a rapid pace. I never treated him like he was going to die; I never treated him with sympathy. I treated him like Larry.

I got it. I hated when people spoke to me like I wasn't myself, and I would not do that to Larry. Many times, he fell asleep as we'd be watching the Yankees game, and I'd nudge him and say, "Get up, old man, Jeter is up," or something like that. I'd sneak him a sip of beer. I treated him like Larry, although I knew where this ship was headed. There were several times I would prod him to get up to watch baseball with me, and he wouldn't move. I was never spooked or scared. If it was his time, I was there for him regardless.

On June 29th, 2014, we brought my children to the hospital to say goodbye to their grandfather. He was still able to articulate thoughts. It was time for the children to see him and communicate with him for the last time, give him a hug and kiss, and take that memory with them for life.

We drove up to Hershey Hospital, and it would be the last time we spent with him where he was coherent. Before Larry passed, he wasn't able to communicate and was a shell of himself. He was not just my father-in-law; he was my cancer partner, my inspiration, and my idol for the way he fought with independence and dignity. We drove up to Rebecca's parents home so we can say goodbye to him. He was incoherent and emaciated. Rebecca said goodbye to him. She was overwhelmed with emotion. I waited for Rebecca to leave the room to have my conversation with Larry. When she left, I let him know I'd never be the man I am, the cancer survivor, or the husband without him. I would always take care of his family, and it was time for him to be with us in a different way.

I believe Larry was waiting for that conversation with his partner, his son-in-law. I saw it in his eyes, which spoke to me when nothing else did. He knew what I said, and he had the comfort he needed. On the next day, July 28, 2014, Larry passed away. I knew he was in a better spot, but it still hurt that he was gone.

What my wife went through brought back memories of my mother dealing with death of my Grandma Harriet. Rebecca would never be the same; she didn't want her dad to go. I didn't either, but I understood. He will never leave us; he just communicates with us in a different way now. Let me make this clear: *cancer did not win.* Larry did. The inspiration he created for his family and the fight he put up, all the while maintaining class and dignity…that will be his story and his legacy. A story of fight, love, and family. Cancer may have ended Larry's time with us earlier than it should have, but it will never end the legacy of the man who was, and still *is,* my partner on my journey and fight with cancer.

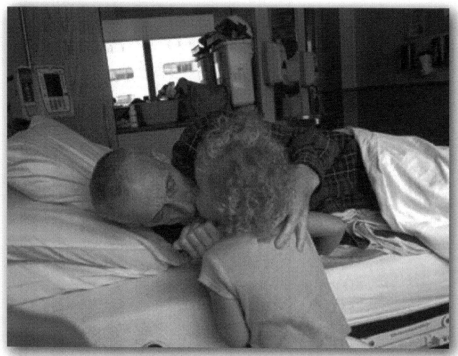

June 29th, 2014. Hershey Hospital with Lola.

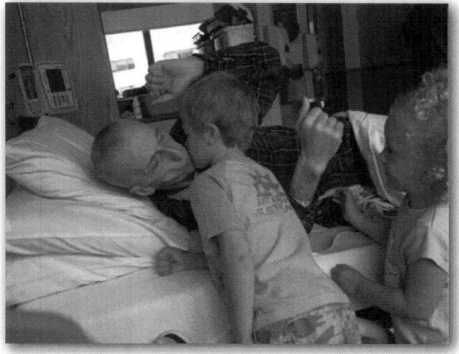

June 29ᵗʰ, 2014. Hershey Hospital with Jake.

In August, 2014, I had my next MRI/MRA. The next day, we met with the group of doctors, and the news they shared was all positive. No cancer had grown back, and they would see us in three months. The news was great, and the relief was enormous, but what I also realized was that the digestion of and decompression from this result was more difficult than it had been in the past. Rebecca needed this news, inside she was a mess. Thinking that after losing her father she can't take hearing that the tumor had grown back, good news was essential. I was happier for her then I was for myself when we received the news we needed to hear. She deserved a moment of reprieve.

I take all experiences I have encountered on my journey and try to capitalize on the knowledge I have taken from them to continually strive to be better at life. My next MRI was three months later in November, and some good things were happening to me. My taste buds had returned. I had succumbed to the fact I would never have them again, and was OK with it. When I started to taste food again, my appreciation of food was at a level that is indescribable. Things were getting better. Lethargy was starting to go away, my stomach was much better and going to the bathroom wasn't the issue it had been. Physically things were heading in the same direction as my perspective. This next test, bring it on, all good news is coming!

This was an MRI that unexpectedly led to nerves, sleepless nights, and more anxiety than usual. I am always strong and know good things will happen, and usually I can deal with these fairly routinely. I was trying to figure out why this one was causing me such angst. I usually do not think about these tests until a day or two before, and then I get extremely amped up to beat them. This time, I was more nervous than before. Why was I feeling this way?

As we drove to the hospital to get my MRI, I realized why. On July 28th, we lost Larry to pancreatic cancer. A forty-nine-month fight had ended, and the grieving for my family had begun. Over the last two-plus months, we all got tighter, and we all mourned. I also saw my wife start to heal. She will never get over losing her father at sixty-four years old, but she seemed to come to peace with it, and the recovery had begun. The last thing I wanted to see was my wife being dealt another blow.

My eighth wedding anniversary would be the following week after the MRI. During a moment of positive reflection, I thought of our family, and life. I was also confronted with a period of negative reflection, and I thought of her father's pancreatic cancer, my brain tumor, prostate surgery on my father, and the loss of her grandmother, my grandmother, and her father. I couldn't have more bad news for her. Her fight, her strength, her inspiration has been undeniable. I am beyond lucky to have such a beautiful, loving, and strong woman by my side. I believe the added nervousness came from the need to provide comfort and stability to my wife, who always provided it to our entire family.

When I received my results, I, of course, was massively relieved. Oddly enough, I didn't have a crazy feeling of happiness, but instead, I was more confused. My family was ecstatic with the news. The doctors would see me in three months, and life would continue to remain the same. I had no side effects, no speech issues, no concerns, and life was normal.

Why was I not overwhelmed with joy? I believe it was because I was so preoccupied worrying about my wife getting good news that I needed time to decompress and digest the results that were given to me. It was so important

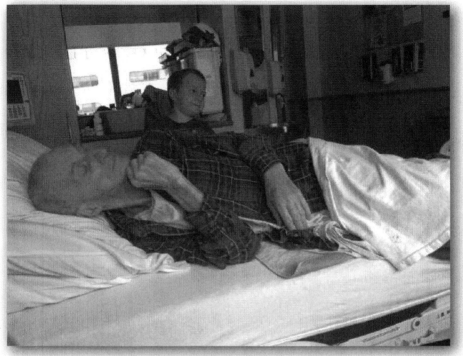

June 29th, 2014. Hershey Hospital with Luke.

for me to allow Rebecca to continue to focus on healing, family, and good things, that as great as the results were, I was taken aback and needed time to understand how good this was.

I don't think they teach this in schools or in bedside manner classes...that sometimes good news is so badly needed and so overwhelming, it's hard to just take it in, smile, and move on. The doctor's talk with us could not have gone better, and I had digested that. This good news allowed me to continue to appreciate life more and more every day. Most importantly, it allowed me to maintain the shift in perspective that makes me a better person.

At the end of 2014, a good friend I work with had sent me an e-mail. I was the top producer at my company again that year. He told me he was honored to be my friend, and that what I was doing both personally and professionally was extremely special. I was really touched by his message. I didn't look at myself as doing anything other then what I was supposed to do. I wrote him back, "Thank you. I appreciate those kind words, but that's not true. I'm just a regular guy who loves his family and refuses to give up." I was just being myself, someone I now understood more. Someone I was at peace with. Someone who wanted to help.

Eighteen

2015 THE NEW NORMAL

The year 2015 was off to an excellent start personally as well as professionally. I felt great and was probably in the best shape of my life physically. I was spending time snowboarding with my six- and seven-year-old boys, and the appreciation of that time together, doing something we all love to do, was something I cherished and will never forget. Seeing my four-year-old daughter dance and get her ears pierced was a beautiful thing to be a part of. Walking my dogs, playing with my kids, and watching them grow is something I looked at in a different light than I did prior to my operation.

March of 2015 was my next MRI. I thought I knew what would happen: I would walk in, get a positive report, and move on. Easy, right? Things aren't always as easy as they sound. With the perspective change that I was gifted with through this terrible disease, I was allowed the opportunity to look at things differently then I did prior to being sick. The job of helping people be prepared for the unexpected, and providing some semblance of good news when they needed to hear it the most was something I looked forward to every day more than ever.

Taking each day one day at a time and appreciating the relationships we have built over the years continues to be a gift that I received from this awful disease. That's right; I believe I was given a gift from cancer. Continuing to focus on what's happening today and living more in the moment is something I worked on and focused on daily. Preparing for what's going to happen tomorrow rather than constantly looking backward and always focusing on what's happened yesterday continued to make me stronger, sharper, and more on point.

I understood that as someone goes through an awful life event, his or her perspective will often change. I believe that if it is handled correctly, it is the gift we are given. We receive it as an opportunity in exchange for going through such a difficult experience. It's a shame you have to go through something terrible to learn some of the greatest lessons life provides.

As I got further away from my operation, which would be two years ago on May 17th, and because awful life events get further away in the rearview mirror for many, I could see how people can resort back to old habits. Constantly working to get better, and using these gifts going forward is difficult. It's work. The further away these life events get from us, the easier it can be to resort to old ways of living, thinking, and acting. The doctor's that operated on me did such wonderful work. You could barely see the scar on the left side of my head. Oddly enough, I wished I could see it. Anytime I would get annoyed, every time I had the desire to go back to old ways, seeing that scar would be a reminder to take a deep breath and remember the lesson that cancer has given me. We can give back these gifts that I look at as a reward for getting through life's toughest challenges. I will always work to make sure I don't let that happen. This gift is mine, it's a victory for me over cancer.

My next MRI was on March 11th, 2015, and was probably the least stressful one I was going to deal with, or so I thought. This would be easy; I would show up, have my MRI, take my tests, get my good news, and be on my way.

It was also that time of year again that I was training for the Broad Street Run where Team Newmanium would raise more money for the National Brain Tumor Society, and all was going well. Why be stressed out? This testing thing would be a cakewalk. I would get a good report and see them again in three months. That's what I thought would happen.

Unfortunately, things don't always go the way we want or expect. On Sunday night, I started to feel anxiety. I did not understand it. I had done this test a bunch of times; I knew the drill, and I felt great; why was I getting all anxious? I also noticed on Sunday night that I was barely able to sleep. My mind was racing. This really had not happened to me before. I kept asking myself what was going on. The more I asked myself, the more nervous and anxious I got.

I went to work Monday; all was good. After work I went to the gym, had a great workout, and figured maybe the previous night was a fluke. On Monday night, I went to sleep at nine thirty; I was going to work all day on Tuesday and get to my MRI by four thirty in Hopewell, New Jersey. I woke up that night, figuring it was about 3:00 or 4:00 a.m., but when I looked at the clock, it was 10:30 p.m.

I slept for an hour, and my mind was still racing. It was happening again. Anxiety was kicking in; nervousness was hitting me. I didn't fall asleep until 3:30 a.m. My mind was all over the place. I kept saying to myself, "I feel great; all the news will be good. Why am I so nervous?" I didn't know why I was, but I was.

I thought this whole thing would be a breeze. But I couldn't sleep, and any free time I had, my mind was continuously racing. It was the most nervous I've been for any cancer testing I have done. I tried everything, and the nerves continued to hit me. After my MRI, I went to dinner with my wife like we do after every MRI. I didn't feel hungry; I felt nervous. I thought maybe a drink would take the edge off, it didn't. I barely slept, and I just focused on seeing the doctors the next day.

My appointment was for 9:00 a.m., but I didn't get any news until almost noon. I had a full day planned, but this appointment ended up monopolizing most of my day. Doctors' schedules are different from those of us in the financial world. We strive to stay on time and maximize our time. I, however, was on a doctor's schedule, which meant he would see me when he would see me.

When Dr. Patchell, our new Oncologist, finally came into our room, he told us no cancer had grown back. "Things look good, and let's keep this great news going." The smile on Rebecca's face was glowing; she was so happy. I smiled briefly, and then my smile went away. All the stress, anxiety, and all that comes along with this test started to release.

My eyes teared up rather than smiling. I looked somber. Was I happy? Of course. But I needed time to decompress and absorb this good news. I understood it was the best news I can get, but it would be revisited in June. It will never be something that goes away. It's part of my life now, and I have to live with it.

Rather than feeling the happiness that Rebecca felt, the happiness that shined all over her face, I felt relief. Shedding the nerves and anxiety was harder than I expected, but when they were finally released, joy set in, joy that I would be here for my children and Rebecca. I will continue to focus on never giving back this unexpected gift I was given for going through cancer, the gift of living for today.

In June of 2015, we had two big events. My mother had her retirement dinner; she was retiring from being an ESL (English as a second language) teacher in her hometown of Fair Lawn, New Jersey. That day, I watched three women retire, reflect, and look forward. Their appreciation for their jobs and their love of the children they taught was really something to behold. They laughed, they cried, and they reflected. They also all talked about their futures: spending time with grandchildren, picking up new hobbies, and doing what they wanted. They praised the security of pension plans and benefits. They all took shots at Chris Christie, which the conservatives in the room chuckled at. It was a celebration of the past and an optimistic look forward.

I was so proud of my mother. She did what she wanted, which was important and satisfying to her, and she had her future to enjoy and fulfill herself. It was an optimistic sendoff. The looking forward and living in the now reminded me of the lessons I have learned from my battle with cancer: living for the moment, focusing on the future, and not spending your time looking backward. I was a very proud son and very determined that I would get great news from my MRI to cap off the week and let my mother know I would be right there with her through retirement.

The second event we had was the kindergarten graduation of my middle child, Jake. He was six years old and so excited. He was growing up and would join his older brother at his school next year to begin first grade. When we got to the graduation, the parents, grandparents, and siblings who came turned out to be a pretty crazy amount of people. We watched the kids get diplomas, sing, and say goodbye to kindergarten.

We saw speeches on what in life was coming next and that the kids would be ready; the teachers showed their appreciation for the children. It was a very emotional week for me. I saw Jake graduate, and I saw my mother retire, yet none of this would be enjoyed or celebrated if bad news came from my MRI. I didn't want this to be about me; I wanted it to be about them.

My fight with cancer and all the baggage it brings to the table would continue. I knew I'd get positive news, but there were always the anxious thoughts. Am I going to get bad news with all these good things happening in my family? Will it now be about pity for me and not happiness for them? I can't get bad news now; I won't get bad news. That was the thought in my head. The reality was that it was out of my control.

On June 10th, 2015 I received my test results back, they showed nothing had grown back. I was happy for my family; I was mostly happy for my mother and Jake. I thank my mother and father for the man I've become. Without their guidance and support, I would never be who I am proud to be today.

I am so proud of all my children, and I thank God every day for them (even when they acted like the crazy four, six, and seven year-olds that they were). This was Jake's day. I spent the balance of the day with my wife. We went to dinner, went to get ice cream, and just talked and laughed. We spoke about all the good in our lives and looked back on a lot of the bad. We saw nothing but positives going forward and were strong enough to deal with the negatives.

We won't sweat the little things, but we will appreciate the moment and the special things that happen on a daily basis. I wake up every morning and look forward to the day ahead. There are days that there are issues, problems, and things that drive me nuts. But through all of it, I do the best I can every day to be the best dad, husband, son, friend, and business partner I can be, and I will never stop having that outlook.

Cancer has given me an ability to have better appreciation and understanding. Heroes are made when they conquer the difficult and rise to the challenge. Anyone can do it when things are easy. When things are hard, my family will get stronger, and our ability to deal with difficult times will make all of us heroes to those around us.

The further along my journey went, the more emotion and raw feeling I poured into my presentations for work. They were mine. Sharing them was paying it forward, releasing my emotions. I was optimistic and, at the same time, always aware of the reality, evilness, and uncertainty of the disease I danced with. I used to push it down and try to not address it or deal with it. My messaging allowed me to own it. I got it, processed it, and dealt with it.

Connecting with others and helping them to plan physically and financially allowed me to have an outlet to unload my emotion. I found my way of showing ownership in what I had and what I dealt with. The deeper I would go, the more calls and messages I would get looking for assistance, looking for a voice. I love the quote from Voltaire and Spiderman, "With great power comes great responsibility." I have the ability to share, and with it, I have a responsibility to be there in mind, body, and spirit when questions are asked of me. I never asked for this job, nor was I interviewed for it. This came with my method of releasing my emotions on others, and I welcomed it.

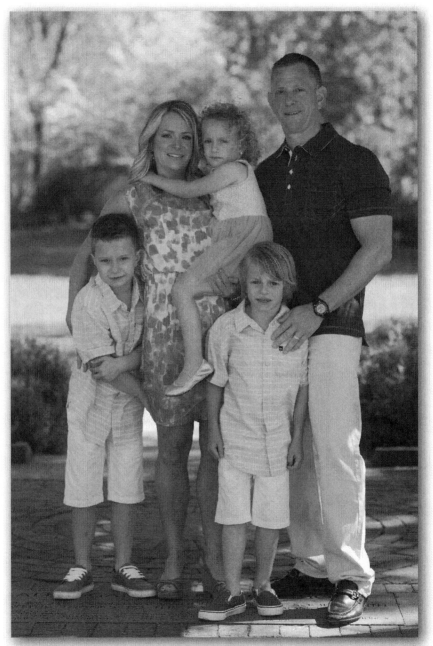

June 20th, 2015. The Art Museum, Philadelphia.

Nineteen

May 14th, 2016 was my third anniversary of being diagnosed with brain cancer. It had been a very different morning than I expected. This day was supposed to be a day of celebration. I felt great! We were raising money for charity to beat this awful disease. On May 1, we ran our third Broad Street Run for charity, and we had raised just about $55,000 to beat brain cancer and support families affected by this awful disease. This was going to be a day of appreciation, a day of celebration, a day of victory. As I continued to learn, things don't always work out the way we want or expect. It had become a day of reflection and consternation.

That morning when I woke up, I was not in the optimistic and excited mood that I usually was. I was sullen and quiet. I was digesting what we have been through for not only the last three years, but throughout life. For some reason, I started processing a retrospective on who we are and where we came from.

I'd been thinking about my Grandma Harriet a lot lately, this day more than ever. Over the past week, I had thought more about her than I have during the last thirty years combined. Why was this on my mind so much now?

I always think of Larry; the bravest man I have ever watched fight a battle. Knowing that my wife had three kids, two dogs, and her husband and father with cancer and undergoing chemotherapy, all in the same house at the same time, always reminds me who the strongest person I know is. Rebecca was burdened unfairly, and she did what needed to be done. Her strength and support were unexplainable.

I miss Larry every day, and that day, I woke up sadder than I had been in a long time that he was not there with me. I wanted us both to beat it. It didn't work out that way. I was thinking of all the people I have met, interacted with, and spoken to who needed encouragement and strength to continue their fight. My emotions began to overcome me with sadness.

Cancer is like buying a new car. When you buy a car, you start to notice that car everywhere. You never really noticed it around that much before, but when you buy it, you tend to see it all over. You become more perceptive to it because you have a connection to it. Cancer is the same. The amount of people I've met, spoken with, and cried with is countless. I was thinking of all those people that day. I was thinking of their families, and my thoughts, prayers, and respect went out to all of them.

This day was supposed to be a day of happiness, a moment of victory for me and my family. I am well aware that with cancer, positive outcomes can change at any time. This was a day to live in the moment and flourish with the family I am privileged to have. A day to smell the roses. The reality is that it didn't feel that way. I was beyond appreciative for those that have surrounded me and helped me fight. They inspired me to never give up. I believe without their support, I would never have the optimism I have, nor would I be in the situation that I am in, which is healthy and thankful.

I was sad thinking about the people who have fought this fight who were no longer there to celebrate with me. I missed them and hated that their lives have been taken by something completely out of their control. I missed my grandmother. I hated that I saw my mom cry so much. I missed my father-in-law. I hated what it did, and still does, to Rebecca. I hated that I was crying while I was writing this.

I hadn't cried out of sadness in a long time, but that was the day that the emotions were pouring out of me. I will never give up trying to beat this disease. This can be beaten, and my life's emphasis, besides family and loved ones, will be to continue to raise money for charities that support research to beat cancer and help the families who are going through this difficult process.

We often feel alone when we go through difficult times. We try to talk to people, and out of kindness and love, they act like they understand. The truth is, if you haven't been through it or dealt with a loved one going through it, you don't understand. I have learned sometimes it's good to just smile, hug, and just let others know you are there. I wish I was more understanding as a child so I could have been there more for my mother. I just didn't understand the ramifications of what was really happening.

Lessons are taught in a variety of different ways. Sometimes the most important ones are delivered at the toughest of times. On this day, I learned that the three-year anniversary of my diagnosis was not a celebration; it was an emotional and hard-to-swallow vision of what led me to where I was that day. I was a better person, husband, father, son, brother, and friend. Going forward, I realized that it was about appreciating what brought me to that point and understanding how it occurred. This was not a day of celebration. It was a day of reflection.

Three years ago, my life changed forever. There are days when it feels like May 14th, 2013, was decades ago, there are days when it feels like it was ten minutes ago. The lessons I have learned have been life altering. Every day, I tried to find the angle to make them positive and inspiring while knowing that to neglect and not acknowledge the negative would be negligent. It would be wrong. I am here for the purpose of appreciating all that I have and all that I've learned and to help in any capacity possible.

My grandmother, my father-in-law, and all of those I've met who aren't with us any longer are a large part of what keeps me fighting. They keep me on point. Knowing what they went through has helped to prepare me for my journey, which is something I never realized until this day. They know my journey is *far* from over. There is more we will do to help, and there is more love to give.

The truth is, my life was not all unicorns and rainbows. I tried to appreciate as much as possible, but we all deal with pain, anger, and sadness. For all of the optimism I've felt, to say there was not difficulty would be untrue. I was connecting with people, those I knew weren't getting any better. Losing those people who I have connected with is painful and has made my hatred of cancer grow more and more.

Cancer taught me lessons, and I looked at those teachings as a gift. The experience I had has allowed me to deal with my sadness, has helped me address my challenges, and has given me the ability to live in the now and share my perspective with others. For all the positives it has taught me, the underbelly is negative. Cancer will not be my legacy. I own my legacy.

Twenty

2017 FOUR YEARS AFTER DIAGNOSIS

My MRIs would now be every four months. More good news. On January 7th, 2017, I had my first MRI after a four-month wait, no longer three months! Even though it had been four months, this time it felt like ages since I had last been in a hospital for my tests. When I walked in the hospital, and the woman behind the desk said, "Hello, Mr. Newman. Time goes by quickly; feels like you were just here." All of a sudden, I felt the same.

It's amazing how thoughts and perspective can change on a dime. I was in the tube for an hour, got out around 6:00 p.m., and my wife and I went out for our usual dinner. It's interesting; everyone thinks the hardest part is sitting in a tube for that long. To me, it's not. To me the hardest part is staying occupied until I get my results the next day around 10:00 a.m. at the hospital. The waiting is the challenge. No matter how great I feel, no matter how confident I am in my health, the waiting is the hardest part.

I usually get up and hit the gym at 5:30 a.m. to take the stress out; this time I spent the morning with my children, getting them ready for school, helping my wife, and trying to stay in the moment. I watched them get into the car, and then I had about an hour to kill before we went to the hospital. I was confident all would go well, but I also was ready for the information right away. I was not overly emotional. I did not feel a need to try to get the stress off my shoulders until something occurred as we entered the hospital.

Rebecca and I pulled in, got out of the car, and walked into the waiting room, ready to check in. They had just changed the check-in system at Capital Health, so I waved hello to the woman who would always take care of me and let me in without waiting in line. Next, we went to the new check-in counter, and I heard a very loud GONG as we stood in line. I knew what that gong was, and the emotions and reality hit me like a ton of bricks. That GONG was part of me, and it brought out emotions. Emotions I was not prepared to encounter. It made me feel appreciation, strength, and humility.

Someone was celebrating getting through radiation. I couldn't see them, but I felt connected to them. They probably didn't know what the future would hold, but I hope they were in the moment and they were celebrating the milestone that they achieved. It brought me to tears again, and it brought out an enormous feeling of accomplishment of being who I am, where I am, and what I have been through.

The news I received from the doctor was what we expected. Nothing was growing back, I should keep doing what I was doing, and he would see me in May, which would be my four-year anniversary of being diagnosed with brain cancer. I never, ever, want to forget what helped me to get to where I am, and I want to try to help as many people as I can. I received great news about my health, and my family could not be any happier. I will always remember hearing that GONG and then remembering what got me here and what helped change my perspective. What helped make me better.

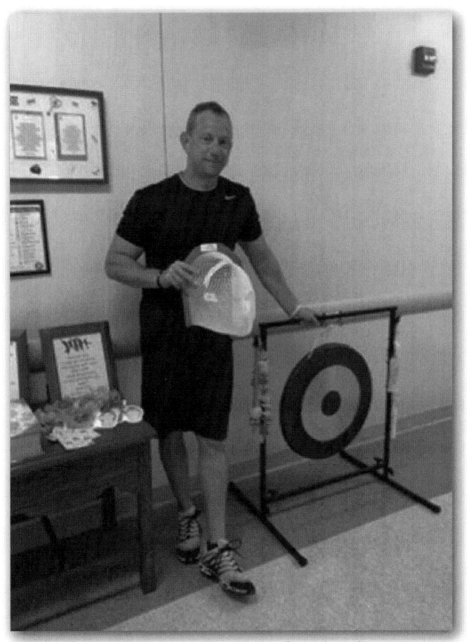

July 14th, 2014. remembering the "Gong" I rang after my last radiation session

Twenty-One

The Final Chapter of a Story that is Far From Over

I was always taught to prepare. My business was based on preparation. I never imagined that all the speeches and meetings I gave, talking about having a plan in place, would actually be about me. My journey with cancer, which is far from over, has taught me lessons I am grateful to have learned. It created a relationship with Larry that I was privileged to be part of. It drove us to a place in our relationship I did not know existed. A place of appreciation, support, and love.

I never thought my emotional perspective would have such a major impact on my life. I never anticipated that planning and healthy living would one day help alleviate the burden of pain and fear that would stem from this awful experience with cancer. Make no mistake about it, I knew I was speaking about the right things to do and the right steps to take, but I never thought they would come into play for my family and me at thirty-nine years old.

These feelings, these emotions, they were mine. We would continue to run races and raise money for charity. May of 2017 marked my four-year anniversary of being diagnosed with brain cancer. We were training for our Broad Street Run in 2017, and our goal was to pass $85,000 in charitable contributions.

On May 16th, 2017, I went in for my MRI/MRA as usual, with every intention of celebrating and appreciating my journey over the last four years. The MRI process often invoked emotions that I didn't expect, sometimes didn't understand, and many times didn't want. Through it all, I focused on receiving good news and continued to try to push the other feelings away.

On this day the MRI seemed longer and more tedious than usual. I knew this was an important day for us, and anxiety had definitely kicked in. As much as I tried to focus on staying positive and as much as I tried envisioning the smile I would see from Rebecca when we were told the good news that I knew was coming, the unease continued to linger.

It was a long hour in the MRI tube. When we got home, I tried my best to sleep, knowing that the next day would bear results on where my journey with cancer would lead me. Despite doing my best maintain my confidence that all was good, I couldn't shake the nerves, and I couldn't help but feel off-kilter as I awaited hearing the results.

When we got to the hospital to check in the next day, my mind started racing, and I became very quiet. Each moment spent waiting for the doctor felt like an eternity. This wasn't just another MRI results appointment; four years was a big deal. When Dr. Patchell opened the door and walked into the room to deliver the results, I looked up with anticipation and concern. He smiled and said all was good for the time being. Decompression time. I felt the weight lift off my shoulders, and I could not wait to share the news with my family. I felt humbled, happy, and extremely appreciative of the time and opportunity I still had ahead of me. This was our moment, one of relief and of thanks. We immediately left the hospital, and all I wanted was to see and hug my kids.

The next day, I was holding an event for eight of my clients outside of Baltimore, and my father was one of them. He picked me up, and we made the two-and-a-half-hour drive together.

It's incredible how perspective shifts during life-altering events. Before my battle with cancer, I probably would have met my father at the meeting. But now, my goal was to spend as much time as I could with my Dad, and a long 2.5-hour ride gave us time to be together and talk.

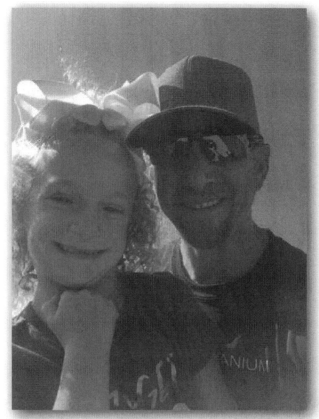

May 17th, 2017. Lola and Daddy celebrating the good news.

The next day after the event we drove back together, and my father wanted to make sure he saw his grandchildren. We got home about 4:55 p.m., and when we walked in the house, my oldest son, Luke, was writhing in pain on the couch. Rebecca told me he was riding his bike to his buddy Billy's house when a truck came flying down the street.

Our neighborhood does not have sidewalks or streetlights. Luke got nervous as the truck was coming and tried to ride onto the side of the road, which is covered in grass and brush. When Luke rode onto the rubble and grass, his handlebars turned and dug under his rib cage as he fell off his bike. Despite being in a lot of pain, he made it a few hundred yards to Billy's house.

Billy's dad immediately drove him home because he was in so much pain. When I got home, I looked at his belly; there were not any cuts, nor were there any bruises. I told him we all fall off our bikes; he would be OK, and there was nothing to worry about.

The next day, Luke was still in a lot of pain but seemed a little better. That night, I was taking Luke, Jake, Billy and my Godson Gavin to the Philadelphia Union soccer game. The kids were so excited, I couldn't wait to spend an evening at a soccer game with my boys and their friends. This day was ours, and I soaked in every second of it.

When we left the game to go home, Luke was walking very slowly and was still in considerable pain. When we got home, he fell right to sleep. Around 4:30 in the morning, he woke up screaming in pain. It had been a few days since Luke fell on his bike, we knew it was time to take him to the hospital. I took him right to Capital Health, the hospital I had grown so familiar with over the years: it was the one I was in when I was diagnosed with cancer, when I went under to be operated on; and when I received the news of being four years cancer free.

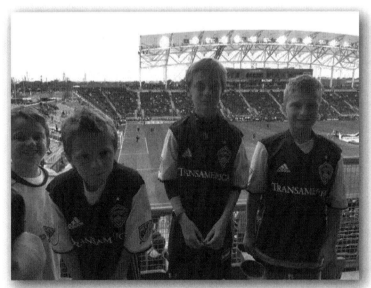

Gavin, Jake, Billy, and Luke at the Philadelphia Union game.

We arrived at the emergency room at about 5:00 a.m., and we were the only people there. I went over every detail with the doctors, and they told me Luke would need a CAT scan to make sure all was OK. Not a problem, I thought. Luke could handle this. Painless and easy. One of the doctors came back a few minutes after the scan and asked if she could talk to me in the other room.

My heart dropped. All I could think was, "Fuck…there is no one else in this hospital. Why do you need to speak to me in the other room?" I knew it was bad immediately.

The doctor looked at me and told me that Luke's liver was nearly split in half, and he needed to be medevacked immediately to CHOP (Children's Hospital of Philadelphia). My heart sank, and fear and anger hit me hard.

My first thought was, "Give me the fucking cancer back. Don't do this to my son!" I immediately called Rebecca and told her she needed to get to the hospital as quickly as possible. She arrived shortly after, and she and Luke got on a helicopter to get down to CHOP. I had to drive and meet them there.

It's a thirty-five-minute ride to CHOP, and my head was all over the place. To see my child being flown to the hospital was the most fear I had ever experienced. We had just received positive news from my tests. Everything was supposed to be good, and yet here we were, fielding another one of life's curve balls.

When I got to the hospital, Luke was in a room with what seemed like twenty people poking and examining him. He was crying in pain and fear. I did everything possible to hold back the tears and be strong for him because that's what he needed most.

When we spoke to the doctor, he told us that the liver is a regenerating organ, and as long as the bile ducts did not get infected, Luke would eventually be OK. We assumed we would be able to take him home and just keep a close eye on him. Then we realized we were heading to the ICU.

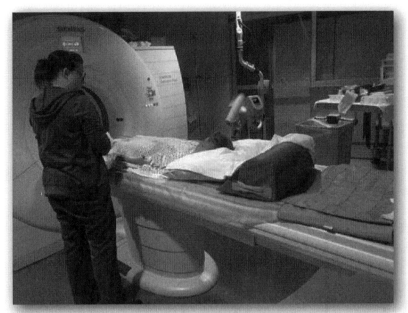

Luke getting a CAT scan.

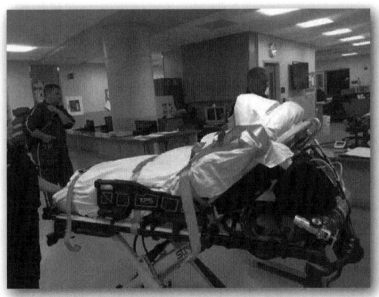

Luke being prepared to be medevacked.

Luke would be in the ICU for two to three days and then remain at CHOP for observation for a day or so. Once we got settled in the ICU, my wife told me that the pilot, a guy named Michael Murphy who flew them down, was extremely helpful to her. He was giving instructions and making sure she was comfortable. Rebecca was extremely scared, and thankful to Michael for all his help. Rebecca took a picture of the helicopter so she would remember him, and was so thankful for the way he helped during such an awful time.

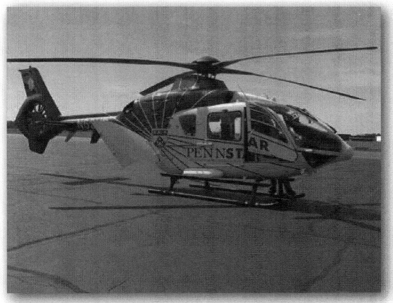

The picture Rebecca took of the helicopter.

Spending time in the ICU at CHOP was beyond humbling. Seeing parents in hazmat suits while they held their newborns was something I had never witnessed. Trying to stay optimistic and positive for Luke was increasingly difficult when we saw what was going on around us. But we knew that as long as Luke did not have an infection, he would eventually be able to go home. We also knew that many families were in a much different situation then we were.

Seeing the strength and composure of so many parents was astonishing to watch, as they focused on embracing the positive, blocking out the negative, and simply being there for their children. What those nurses and doctors do and see on a daily basis in that hospital is absolutely awe-inspiring. To refrain from letting emotion cloud perspective and go on to save a child's life is something that does not get the due it deserves. They are selfless heroes, and it was life-changing to witness these heroes in action. I hope I never see the inside of the ICU again, but it was heroic to see what these medical professionals and parents endured to be there to support and to help when it was truly needed.

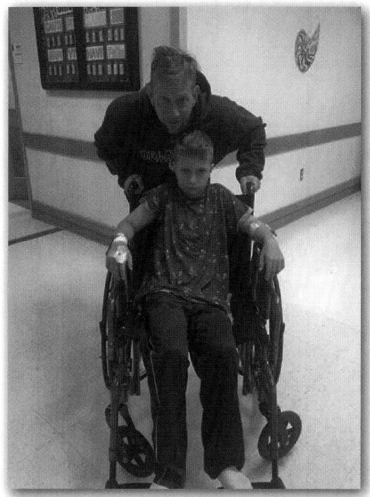

Luke at CHOP in Philadelphia.

On Wednesday, after four long days in the hospital, we were cleared to leave. Luke was not allowed to play contact sports, wrestle around with his brother or sister, or do anything that could potentially cause his liver to start bleeding again. He was required to be very low-key for twelve weeks. Knowing Luke was cleared to leave and knowing that after twelve weeks he would be himself again provided immense relief and happiness to Rebecca and me. It also brought on more sympathy and love for those who were still at CHOP and who hadn't been able to come home. I think about them often, and those memories will always be on my mind.

The next day I was back at work, and Rebecca was watching Luke at home. I received a text from her that day telling me she couldn't stop crying. I immediately called her and asked what was wrong. She asked if I was watching TV, and I told her I was in my car headed to an appointment. I asked her what was going on, and she replied with news that I was not at all prepared to hear.

Rebecca told me that the exact same helicopter that she took a picture of, the one that she and Luke were flown to CHOP in, had just crashed near New Castle County Airport in Delaware. The same helicopter! She was crying, hoping, and praying that Michael Murphy was not on board.

As the news trickled out over the next few days, we found out that thirty-seven-year-old Michael Murphy was the pilot. The report we found online indicated that Murphy "declared a missed approach" and climbed to a higher altitude. The helicopter then turned to the right and descended rapidly before radar contact was lost. The chopper crashed less than a mile from the airport and burst into flames.

Michael died at the scene. We later learned that Michael had a two-year-old child and a pregnant wife. Tears welled, and lives were changed forever. This person, who my wife was so thankful to for taking care of Luke during such a scary experience, was gone. This was the same helicopter my wife and child were on five days earlier.

The news of Michael's accident hit close to home in so many different ways and was a stark reminder to appreciate the moment. Life brings on unexpected changes and challenges, and often there is little we can do about it. In the uncontrolled and unpredictable cadence of life, all we can control is our perspective and our focus. All we can control is living in the now.

What was supposed to be a week of celebration after I heard the results of my MRI took a drastic turn. The good news I received was supposed to trigger a domino effect of only positive things to come, not the opposite. My son's experience in the ICU and Michael losing his life so shortly after helping save Luke served only to heighten my realization that life truly can change in the blink of an eye and that preparation and proper planning are not optional; they are essential.

My four-year relationship with cancer has taken me to many different depths emotionally and physically. It has taken me places I didn't know existed. It has taught me about faith. It has shown me where strength and inspiration lie in each and every one of us and how to deal with seemingly insurmountable difficulty and adversity. Cancer has shown me fear and taught me how to be optimistic at even the toughest of times. It has shown me sorrow.

The relationship I have with cancer will not end. It will forever be a part of my life's journey, whether I like it or not. But I will use my journey with cancer to be better. I will use it to continue to think positively and eliminate negativity. Cancer will never crush my optimism or my strength, nor will it define my legacy. Cancer will be part of my life, and I will continually fight to help beat this disease.

Cancer has given me the gift of a change in perspective. It has given me the gift of truly learning how to live in the moment and appreciate the now, lessons that I am not sure I would have learned without fighting the battle that I have fought.

Many people receive this gift, but their health deteriorates before they can truly appreciate it. I thought I was writing this book for me, when as it turns out I was really writing it in honor all those who have fought this disease.

I was inspired by the memories of Grandma Harriet and Larry. I wrote this for my family. I wrote this for all the families that have dealt with the ramifications of this awful disease. We will beat it and find ways to cure it and prevent it in the future. I hope to be there the day it happens. If I'm not there physically, I will be there spiritually.

The disease will never win, and it will never be what we are remembered for. Our persistent fight and our boundless love will be our legacies, not the cancer. Cancer, you took my grandmother. You took my father-in-law. But you will never take the memories we have of them, and you will never take the love that we will forever have for them.

Cancer; *You may dictate how long we are on this earth, but you will never dictate the legacies we leave.*

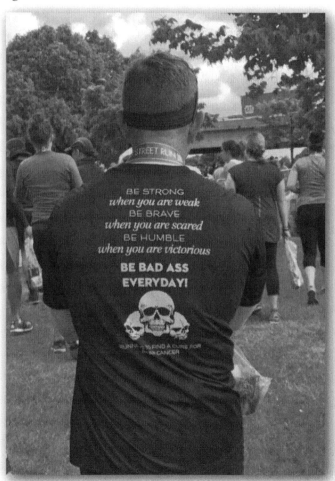

2017 Broad Street Run. Running to beat brain cancer!

81764669R00080

Made in the USA
Middletown, DE
27 July 2018